Did you know . . .

- that in one study, participants were shown photos of two women—and the one with good posture was consistently judged younger and more attractive, even though she was older than the other . . . and twenty pounds heavier?

- that poor posture is the primary cause of back pain—and can also be responsible for neck pain, leg pain, headaches, and other chronic physical symptoms?

- that good posture can improve breathing capacity and athletic performance?

- that your posture has a big impact on how others see you—and how you see yourself?

With *Posture, Get It Straight!* you can discover the dramatic and surprising benefits of improved posture—and take a stand for better health!

Posture, Get It Straight!

Janice Novak

Illustrated by Barbara A. Beshoar

Produced by Alison Brown Cerier Book Development, Inc.

A PERIGEE BOOK

To order a video demonstrating the exercises and stretches in this book—plus an exercise band—send your name and address and a check for $29.95, plus $4.00 shipping, to: Janice Novak, Inc., P.O. Box 241, Chanhassen, MN 55317. You can also order with a major credit card; send your credit-card number, the expiration date, and your signature. E-mail orders to: fitnovak@aol.com

A Perigee Book
Published by The Berkley Publishing Group
A division of Penguin Putnam Inc.
375 Hudson Street,
New York, New York 10014

Copyright © 1999 by Alison Brown Cerier Book Development, Inc., and Janice Novak
Book design by Lisa Stokes
Cover design by Elizabeth Sheehan
Interior and cover illustrations by Barbara A. Beshoar
Author photo by Glamour Shots® of Minnetonka, Minnesota

First edition: May 1999

Published simultaneously in Canada.

The Penguin Putnam Inc. World Wide Web site address is
http://www.penguinputnam.com

Library of Congress Cataloging-in-Publication Data

Novak, Janice S., 1954–
    Posture, get it straight! / Janice Novak.
        p.   cm.
    ISBN 0-399-52500-9
    1. Posture—Popular works.   2. Posture disorders—Exercise
therapy—Popular works.   I. Title.
    RA781.5.N68   1999
    613.7'8—dc21   98–51991
                                                                                      CIP

Printed in the United States of America

10   9   8   7   6   5   4   3   2   1

To my husband, Rich, and daughters Kate and Rachael. They keep me on my toes and make my life complete.

Acknowledgments

I am eternally grateful to all of the wonderful teachers from whom I've had the privilege of learning. I'd like to thank all the people who've participated in my classes and workshops; I've learned much from their questions and experiences. I'd also like to thank Alison Brown Cerier, who has been a delight to work with and who has undoubtedly helped make this a better book. Thanks also to physical therapist Julie Shanabrook for reviewing the manuscript.

Contents

1

Standing Tall

What Good Posture Can Do for You

- Do you think you would look better if you could just lose ten pounds?

- Are you plagued by back pain? A sore neck? Headaches?

- Have you been shocked by how "rounded over" you look in photographs?

- Do you think you look older than your years, and would love to look ten years younger?

If you answered "yes" to any of these questions, you can make a big difference in your health and your appearance by simply improving your posture.

When you were a child or a teen, was your mother always telling you to "straighten up"? She meant well, of course, but just "straightening up" is not the answer. When most people try to improve their posture, they jam their shoulders back, suck in their tummies, and stand stiff as soldiers. This is wrong not only because no one can sustain the position for more than a few seconds, but also because it does not align the body properly. The position looks and feels unnatural and uncomfortable.

For more than fifteen years, I have taught workshops to help people align their bodies quickly and naturally. My program is not a drug, surgical procedure, alternative therapy, or magic spell, but a combination of easy exercises and practical tips for better posture. The results are both immediate and lasting.

I'm often asked, "After years of bad posture, is there any hope for me?" My answer is always an enthusiastic *yes!* No matter how bad your posture is at this moment, you can turn things around with little difficulty. You can start having better posture not in months, weeks, or even days, but in minutes. You can learn simple exercises that strengthen and stretch the muscles that support good posture and make your new posture a permanent part of your life. If you spend even a few minutes a day, you'll see a big change in only three weeks.

If you're not happy with your posture, you have a lot of company. Bad posture is so common because many of us sit too much, exercise too little, and have habits like hanging our heads forward over our desks and always carrying our ten-ton purses and briefcases on the same side.

I became interested in posture improvement in an effort to help myself. My problems started when I was fifteen. Already tall for my age, I grew four inches that summer, reaching a gangly height of five foot nine. All of my friends, and of course most of the boys, were several inches shorter. Trying not to stick out in the crowd, I stooped. I was literally folding myself over to fit in.

When I was nineteen, a friend gave me several pictures of myself taken at a party. I couldn't believe how round-shouldered I'd become and how dreadful it looked. The damage I'd done to myself really hit home. By this age, I wasn't feeling self-conscious about being tall, so I began a journey to discover whether and how I could undo the damage and reclaim my stature. I studied anatomy and physiology. I got a bachelor's degree in health education, then a master's degree in physical education.

After figuring things out for myself, I discovered that a lot of other people also wanted to look and feel better. I began teaching posture classes and workshops, and soon had a waiting list of interested people. Each year, I lead about a hundred workshops at hospitals, health clubs, and community education programs. I also do special workshops for pregnant women and women who have osteoporosis, and work with individual clients.

My program approaches posture improvement in three ways: alignment, easy exercises to strengthen and stretch, and small but powerful changes in everyday habits like how you sit, sleep, and lift things. The tips, techniques, and exercises can easily be fit into your daily activities, without having to set aside a special chunk of time. Learn the exercises and then do a few here and there throughout your day. In no time at all, you'll be reaping the many benefits of standing tall. For inspiration, let's start by taking a closer look at those benefits.

Look Ten Pounds Thinner

Simply by standing straight, you will instantly slim your waistline by an inch or more. Check it out! Place a cloth measuring tape around your waist. Stand your usual way—pretend you're waiting for a bus or an elevator. Now lift up your rib cage slightly, as if a string attached to your breastbone were pulling it toward the ceiling. Check the tape to see how much smaller your waist is. You'll be pleasantly surprised.

(Here's the anatomical explanation for this seemingly magical change: When the upper back slumps forward, it presses the rib cage down on the abdominal organs. The belly protrudes, making the waistline appear larger than it really is.)

Look Ten Years Younger

A study in Louisville, Kentucky, showed how posture affects perceptions of age and beauty. Two women, both five foot four, one weighing 105 pounds and the other 125, were asked to put on leotards and cover their faces. Side-view pictures were taken of each woman with normal and slumping posture. Then sixty people were asked to look at the pictures and rate the women's appearances. When the women stood up straight, viewers consistently described them as younger and more attractive. In fact, the upright 125-pound woman was rated more favorably than the slumping 105-pound woman.

Nothing ages you faster than a shrinking, stooped posture. A strong, straight spine portrays youth and vigor. Slumping forward decreases your chest measurement, causes rounded and narrow shoulders, and can even cost you as much as two inches in height.

Radiate Confidence

Psychological studies have shown that good posture exudes health, vitality, and confidence, while slouching signals insecurity, weakness, and self-doubt. Consciously or not, we tell the world a lot about our mental and emotional state by the way we stand, sit, and move. In fact, posture is one of the first three things people notice about each other (the other two are hair and eyes).

Improving your posture can help you build self-esteem, interview well for jobs, improve your work performance (particularly in sales or business), or find a new romantic partner or friends.

Improve Your Athletic Performance

When you work out or play sports, poor posture increases the chance that you will injure your neck, shoulder, upper back, lower back, hips, and knees. Good posture reduces injuries, muscle strain, and aches; helps you move more easily, gracefully, and powerfully; and gives your lungs more room so you have a greater breathing capacity.

Prevent Back Pain

Most important, good posture can prevent a lifetime of annoying and painful back problems. *Poor posture is the leading cause of back pain.*

The spine, or backbone, is the main supporting structure of the entire body. It is composed of twenty-four interlocking bones called vertebrae, which are stacked one upon the other. In between the vertebrae are disks. This is a delicate, finely balanced structure that can easily be injured. When posture is poor, the joints no longer line up the way they're supposed to. Even everyday activities cause them to press into one another, resulting in friction, pain, irritation, and wear.

When the spine is lined up correctly, the muscle groups that support it are in balance. When the slight natural curves in the spine become exaggerated, some muscles are stretched all the time; these muscles become weak. Other muscles are contracted all the time; these become tight. Some muscles are working too hard, others not hard enough. Gradually, the muscles lose their ability to support the body correctly, and posture grows even worse.

If the lower back arches too much, pressure on the joints and the nerves that pass between them can cause dull aches or stabbing, burning pain anywhere from the waist to the tip of the big toe. A head that hangs forward even slightly exaggerates the curve in the upper part of the spine and can cause chronic back pain, a stiff or sore neck, or tingling or numbness in the arms and hands. The head-forward position is also a common cause of tension headaches, the most common kind of headache.

Knowing the basics of good posture can make the difference between a healthy back and an aching one. When properly aligned, your body moves with ease and comfort. The muscles in the front and back of your body work together harmoniously.

Whenever I do a workshop, I feel deeply satisfied and excited as the participants see immediate improvement. I'm happy that you, too, are ready to do something wonderful for your health and happiness.

t w o

Great Posture
Today and Forever

L et's start by looking at good posture, poor posture, and *your* posture. If you're not happy with your "before," don't worry—you will stand straighter this very day.

How Does Your Posture Measure Up?

Start by taking a good look at the way you usually stand, either by having a friend take a side-view picture or by standing sideways in front of a full-length mirror.

- Does your head protrude forward?

- Is your upper back hunched forward in a rounded curve?

- Do your shoulder blades stick out?

- Do your shoulders round over and fall forward?

- Are your shoulders tensed and held up closely to your ears?

- Is your abdomen protruding forward into a potbelly?

- Is your lower back arched or swayed?

- Are your knees locked back?

- Do your ankles roll in, causing your arches to flatten?

These are all common posture problems.

Now remove your shoes and stand with your back against a wall. Place your feet about six inches away from the wall, and hip-width apart.

- Is there a big gap between your lower back and the wall?

- Is there a gap between the back of your neck and the wall?

- Can you not get the backs of your shoulders to touch the wall?

- Can you not touch the back of your head to the wall without arching your neck?

Again, all of these are posture problems.

What Is Good Posture?

When you are standing correctly:

- Your ear, shoulder, and hip are in a straight line from a side view.

- Your head is directly on top of your shoulders.

- Your upper back is fairly straight (not slouched).

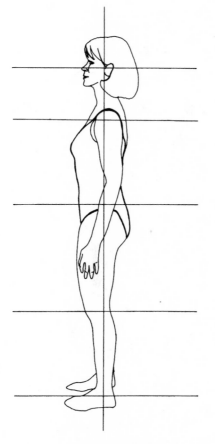

- Your shoulder blades are lying flat against your back.

- Your shoulders are straight and relaxed.

- Your pelvis is in a neutral position (see sidebar on page 12).

- Your knees are unlocked.

Good standing posture

When you sit, you want to maintain the natural curves of your spine. You are sitting correctly when:

- Your ear, shoulder, and hip are in a straight line.

- Your head is centered over your shoulders, not dropped forward.

- Your rib cage is lifted.

- Your arms are supported by armrests.

- Your shoulders are relaxed.

- Your bottom is against the back of the chair.

- Your pelvis is in neutral.

- Your thighs are fully supported by the chair seat.

- Your feet are flat on the floor or a stool.

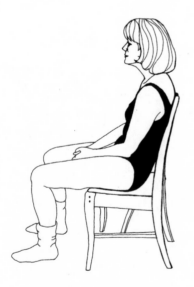

Bad sitting posture

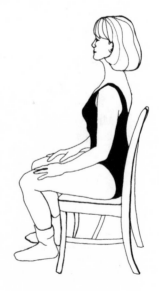

Good sitting posture

Instant Improvement

Don't despair if you don't like the way your posture measured up. There's lots you can do to improve your posture right this very minute. Here's how:

One Minute to Better Posture

Instantly aligns your body.

1. Stand with your feet hip-width apart. Your knees should be soft and neutral, not locked.

2. Pull in your abdominal muscles as if you're zipping up a tight pair of pants. Think of pulling your belly button toward your back.

3. Now you're ready for the most dramatic change. Lift your rib cage up as if there were a string connected from your breastbone to the ceiling, pulling you up. Try to elongate your midsection by pulling your rib cage away from your hipbones.

4. Unround your shoulders by rotating your arms until your thumbs are in a hitchhiking position. Gently press your shoulders down, away from your ears. Pull your shoulder blades toward your spine. Then, without letting your shoulders roll forward, relax your arms. Your palms should end up facing your thighs, and your thumbs should end up pointing straight ahead.

5. Finally, stretch the top of your head toward the ceiling as if a string were pulling you upward.

6. Keep the position for a few moments, trying to relax into it and breathing normally. Then shake yourself a bit, walk around the room for a few minutes, and go through the steps again. The more you practice this, the more comfortable and natural it will feel.

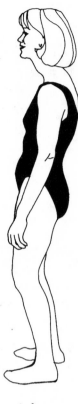

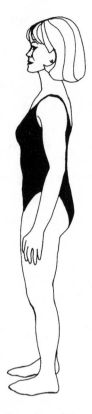

Before   One minute later

One Minute to Better Posture puts the ear, shoulder, and hip in a direct line. Some people with very accentuated spinal curves may need to practice for a while before achieving a direct line between the joints. Every time you do the steps, you will strengthen the muscles of your shoulders, back, and abdomen and teach your body the feel of good posture.

At first, the new position will feel a bit awkward. You're asking your body to behave very differently. But it will not take long to retrain your muscles. If you practice the steps several times a day, in a couple of weeks the position will start to feel natural and really good.

It's useful and interesting to know how each step helps your posture. Let's go through the steps again, this time with a full explanation.

1. **Stand with your feet hip-width apart. Your knees should be soft and neutral, not locked.** Keeping your feet hip-width apart improves your balance and better aligns the feet, knees, and hips. Locking your knees jams your pelvis forward, causing your lower back to sway and your abdominals to stretch and weaken. Over time, it causes wear and tear on the back of the kneecap and can lead to sore knees.

2. **Pull in your abdominal muscles as if you're zipping up a tight pair of pants.** There are four layers of abdominal muscles (abs), each with fibers running in a different direction: horizontal, slanted from right to left, slanted from left to right, and vertical. When the abdominal muscles are strong and toned, this crisscrossed pattern provides tremendous support for the midsection. Strong abs are your core. They support your lower back and help keep everything in place. Also, because the abdominals are attached to the bottom of your rib cage, when you consciously pull them in, you should actually feel the bottom of your rib cage pull in slightly, decreasing your waistline measurement. If you don't feel the bottom of your rib cage pull in, try this. Place your fingertips on your midsection between your rib cage and hipbones. Inhale. As you exhale, pull your belly button into your spine. As you continue to exhale, tap or poke the muscles under your fingertips. Poking the muscles will cause them to contract a bit. Within two weeks, you'll probably be able to tighten those fibers without poking them.

3. **Lift your rib cage up as if there were a string connected from your breastbone to the ceiling. Try to elongate your midsection by pulling your rib cage away from your hipbones.** This simple move makes the biggest difference in your appearance. By decreasing the pressure on your abdomen, it will reduce your waist measurement by an inch or more! It also helps straighten a rounded upper back and gives your lungs more space so you can breathe more deeply. Finally, it helps realign your head over your shoulders. When you

lift your rib cage, be careful that you do not lean backward, which would arch the lower back or bow your chest forward.

4. **Unround your shoulders by rotating your arms until your thumbs are in a hitchhiking position. Gently press your shoulders down, away from your ears. Pull your shoulder blades toward your spine. Then, without letting your shoulders roll forward, relax your arms. Your palms will end up facing your thighs, and your thumbs should be pointing straight ahead.** This repositioning movement is the cure for rounded shoulders. It realigns all the joints in the shoulders. These moves will also give your shoulders their natural width. Your lungs and heart will have more room, too. Also, by positioning your shoulders correctly, you will take a lot of strain off the muscle at the back and side of your neck (the upper trapezius) and will make the muscles of the mid-back begin to do their share of the work.

5. **Finally, stretch the top of your head toward the ceiling as if a string were pulling you upward.** By doing this, you can restore as much as two inches of your natural height! Slumping decreases your height because it exaggerates the curves of your spine. When you stand tall, the spine straightens and you regain your height.

Go through the above steps, then check yourself out in the mirror. Try out your new appearance on your family or friends. They'll see a big improvement. You'll see a big improvement, too, and you'll feel great about yourself. Not only will you look better, but you'll feel better, because your body will be held upright by the muscles designed for that purpose.

> **One, Two, Three, Better Alignment**
>
> Every time you catch yourself slumping:
> 1. Pull in your abdominal muscles.
> 2. Lift your rib cage.
> 3. Unround your shoulders.

For Lasting Change

Now you know what good posture feels like! However, if you've been holding yourself incorrectly for years, your muscles won't be able to keep you aligned properly unless you think about your posture all day long. The trick is to strengthen the muscles that have become too weak, and stretch the muscles that have become too tight, so they will do the work for you.

Here are some easy exercises that will do just that. If you set aside a few minutes each day to do them, you'll see a big change in just a few weeks. After each strengthening exercise, do one of the two stretches (described at the end) to relax the muscles of your back and shoulders. You don't need to change into exercise gear, but you'll feel more comfortable in loose-fitting clothing in which you can bend. All of these exercises will reinforce overall good posture.

Posture Press

Strengthens the mid-back and the back of the shoulders, and reinforces good alignment.

1. Lie on your back, knees bent and feet flat on the floor. Place your arms by your sides, palms facing up, shoulders relaxed. Gently press your shoulders away from your ears, as if you were trying to elongate your neck.

2. Take a deep breath. As you exhale, tighten your abdominals and *gently* press your lower back toward the floor until your pelvis is in neutral. Next, press your middle back, then upper back, into the floor. Now gently press the back of your neck into the floor. Don't force it; just ease your back as close to the floor as is comfortable. You should feel your whole back pressing gently into the floor.

3. Next, press the back of your shoulders into the floor, as if you were trying to press your shoulder blades together. Don't let your lower back come off the floor. You should feel a tightening of all the muscles in your mid-back, and particularly the muscles between and around your shoulder blades. Hold this position for a count of ten. Do not hold your breath. Relax.

4. Repeat several times.

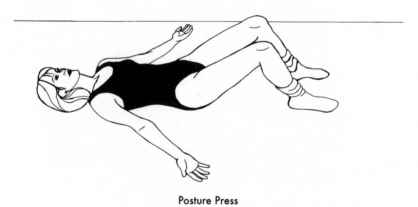

Posture Press

Triangle Press

Strengthens the muscles of the back, shoulders, and abdomen; stretches the front of the shoulders and chest.

1. Lie on the floor with your knees bent and your feet flat on the floor. Clasp your hands behind your head. Press your shoulders away from your ears.

2. Inhale. As you exhale, tighten your abdominal muscles and gently press your lower back toward the floor until your pelvis is in a neutral position. Keep the abs pulled in as tightly as possible. Then press the mid- and upper back into the floor. Gently coax the back of your neck as close to the floor as is comfortable. Don't force it.

3. Next, press your arms and elbows into the floor. Hold the position for a slow count of ten. You'll feel the muscles between the shoulder blades tighten and strengthen.

4. Relax, and then repeat several times.

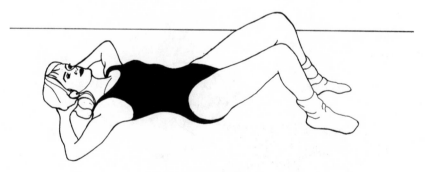

Triangle Press

Angel Wings

Strengthens middle and upper back and abdominals; promotes proper alignment.

1. Lie on your back with your knees and feet turned outward. Keep your heels together.

2. Place your arms by your sides, palms facing up.

3. Inhale. As you exhale, squeeze your buttock muscles and tighten your abdominals, which will press the lower back toward the floor.

4. Without relaxing the abdominal or buttock muscles, slide your arms slowly away from your body along the floor toward your head. *Do not let any part of your back come off the floor.* Some people can slide their arms all the way to their ears while keeping their backs pressed onto the floor; others to shoulder level. Work at your own level. Gradually you will be able to slide your arms further and further.

5. Keeping your back pressed into the floor and your buttocks and abdominals tight, slowly slide your arms back down toward your sides as far as you can while keeping your back flat to the floor.

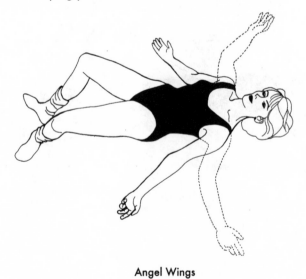

Angel Wings

Wall Press

Helps align your spine.

1. Stand with your back against a wall. Place your heels about six inches away from the wall. Let your arms hang by your sides with your palms facing forward.

2. Bend your knees slightly and press the small of your back against the wall. Bring your lower back as close to the wall as is comfortable until your pelvis is in neutral.

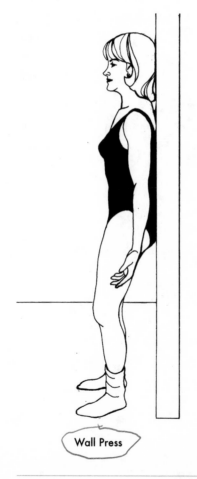

Wall Press

3. Lift your rib cage and press the back of your head to the wall. Bring the back of your neck as close to the wall as is comfortable. Don't worry if there is still a lot of space between your neck and the wall.

4. Press the back of your shoulders into the wall and try to squeeze your shoulder blades as close together as possible. You should feel the muscles tighten in the mid-back and shoulder-blade area. Hold for a slow count of ten, then release.

5. Press your back and both shoulders to the wall. Let your knees bend and slide down the wall as far as it is comfortable for you, maintaining contact between your back and the wall. Slide back up the wall. Relax and repeat. If you feel any discomfort in your knees, don't slide so far down. Make sure you are on a non-slip surface.

Middle-Back Relaxer

Relaxes muscles in the middle and upper back.

1. Lie on your back, knees bent and feet flat on the floor. Clasp your hands and stretch your arms up toward the ceiling.

2. Move your arms in a big, easy circle. Allow your elbows to bend naturally. Circle five times in one direction and five times in the other. This movement should feel good because it gently stretches and relaxes the soft tissue in the mid-back and gently massages the joint linings.

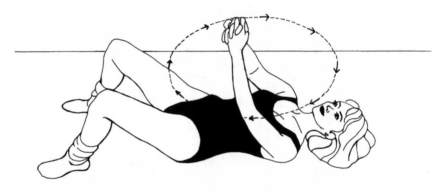

Middle-Back Relaxer

Spine Stretch

Stretches the length of the spine.

1. Lie on your back, knees bent and feet flat on the floor. Stretch your arms behind your head and clasp your hands.

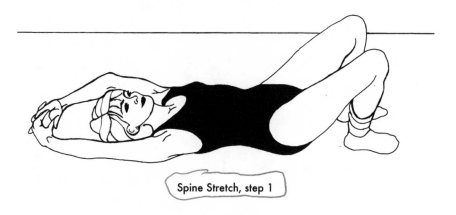

Spine Stretch, step 1

2. Clasping your right knee with your hands, pull it toward your chest. At the same time, pull your head toward your chest. Hold for a few seconds. You'll feel a good stretch down the length of your spine.

3. Uncurl and lie flat on the floor again. Alternate knees.

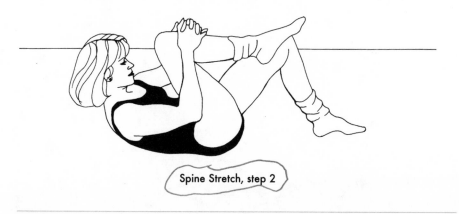

Spine Stretch, step 2

t h r e e

Your Posture Program

N ow that you know several exercises for overall good posture, you can use the *One Minute to Better Posture* every time you catch yourself slumping or letting your head hang forward. Every time you realign yourself, you'll retrain your body. You've also identified your trouble spots, so you'll know where to focus.

It's time to think about ways you can fit your posture work into your already busy life. I think the most effective and practical approach has three parts: practicing good posture throughout the day, fitting in some anytime/anywhere exercises, and setting aside a few minutes each day for posture work (especially for the first three weeks).

Part 1: Practicing Good Posture

The most important way to improve your posture is simply to stay properly aligned as much as possible. Every time you consciously align your body, you reinforce good posture. Do the *One Minute to Better Posture* exercise often, particularly in the first weeks. Also, practice good posture when you're standing, sitting, driving, working, even sleeping (in part 3, you'll find easy tips). If you were to exercise one hour each day, but had poor posture for the other twenty-three hours, your body would continue its bad habits. To receive the full benefit of this program, try to work as many exercises and positioning techniques as possible into your daily life.

Part 2: Anytime/Anywhere Exercises

The second part of the program is to make a habit of anytime/anywhere exercises. These simple, inconspicuous, relaxing moves require no change of clothes, no loss of time, and no perspiration. They can be done whenever you have a few moments: waiting at a red light or elevator, working at your desk or computer, talking on the phone, cooking, and so on. The more often you do them, the better and faster the results will be. These easy exercises will teach your body to recognize proper alignment, strengthen and stretch important muscles, and help you look and feel better.

Try to do them often throughout your day, especially the ones that focus on your particular posture problems. It is better to fit the anywhere/anytime exercises into your day, and realign yourself every time you catch yourself slumping, than it would be to set aside chunks of time several times a week to exercise (which, let's face it, most of us never do). You'll be amazed how much exercise you can fit into your daily routine.

- Do the *Neck Glide* (page 38) every time you catch yourself with your head hanging forward.

- If you are sitting at a desk or computer, take breaks for the *Shoulder-Blade Squeeze* (page 53), *Back Lift* (page 103),

Shoulder Unrounder (page 50), and *Elbow Press* (page 51). Whenever you feel neck or shoulder or back discomfort, these exercises will help relieve it.

- If you have a sway back, potbelly, or lower-back discomfort, do *Abdomen Tighteners 1* and *2* (pages 68, 69). They are inconspicuous and can and should be done every time you think of it. Also, do the *Buttock Clencher* (page 70) often (it's inconspicuous, too).

- *Exhale and Relax* (page 102) will relieve tension in any muscle group.

- Do the *Stretch and Grow* (page 102) whenever you get up from your desk. It'll feel fabulous and will make your midsection appear thinner.

- Do a *Wall Press* (page 21) while you're talking on the phone or waiting for an elevator.

- To help flatten the upper back, do ten *Wall Push-Ups* (page 45) before leaving for work, and upon returning home.

- To help unround your shoulders, do the *Door Frame Stretch* (page 54) for ten to twenty seconds every time you pass through a door.

- For a total spine stretch, do the *Sink Stretch* (page 67) whenever you find yourself at a sink: after brushing your teeth, washing dishes, or taking vitamins.

Part 3: Posture Exercises

For the first three weeks, set aside about ten minutes a day for posture exercises that will strengthen and stretch your muscles.

Week 1

- Practice the *One Minute to Better Posture*.

- Spend 5 minutes a day on the following all-over posture improvement exercises from chapter 2: *Posture Press, Triangle Press, Angel Wings,* and *Wall Press.*

- Do the *Pelvic Tilt for Beginners* (page 61) several times a day.

- Do *Ab Stabilizer, Level 1* (page 63).

- Do the *Hitchhiker* (page 49) several times a day.

- Fit in as many anytime/anywhere exercises as you can each day, especially the *Abdomen Tighteners 1* and *2* (pages 68, 69) and the *Shoulder Unrounder* (page 50).

- Adjust your car seat and headrest (see chapter 11). Drive with good posture.

- If you work in an office, rearrange your workstation to make it more back-friendly, as described in chapter 10.

- Make adjustments to your sleeping position with pillows (see chapter 12).

Week 2

- Continue using the *One Minute to Better Posture* every time you catch yourself slumping.

- Continue to sprinkle in the anywhere/anytime exercises, making sure you do the *Abdomen Tighteners* at least several times each day.

- Continue with the all-over posture improvers.

- Do *Ab Stabilizers, Levels 1* and *2.*

- Graduate to the *Pelvic Tilt, Intermediate Level* (page 61).

- Do the *Middle-Back Relaxer* (page 22) or *Spine Stretch* (page 23) between specific posture exercises.

- Do the *Sink Stretch* (page 67) once in the A.M. and once in the P.M.

- Spend five to ten minutes doing exercises for one specific posture problem. To unround your shoulders, do the *Elbow Press* (page 51), *Goal Post* (page 52), *Door Frame Stretch* (page 54), and *Shoulder Unrounder* (page 50). To flatten your upper back, do the *Upper Back Arch* (page 46), *Wall Push-Up* (page 45), *Wall Press* (page 21), *Triangle Press* (page 19), and *Middle-Back Relaxer* (page 22). If you are often in the head-forward position, do *Putting Your Head in Its Place* (page 38), *Neck Straightener* (page 39), and *Trap Stretch* (page 40). To decrease a sway back, do *Ab Stabilizers* (pages 63–64), *Pelvic Tilts* (pages 61–62), and *Rock and Roll* (page 66).

Week 3

- Continue all of the above.

- Add a second focus for specific posture exercises (if you've been working on your shoulders but also have a sway back, add back exercises now).

After Week 3

After three weeks, you will definitely see improvement. Here are some ways you can continue your program. Stick with the anytime/anywhere exercises and the good posture habits, too.

- If you work out or play a sport, include a few of your favorite posture exercises when you're doing other strengthening or stretching moves.

- In part 2, explore other exercises for your personal posture problems, to keep things interesting.

- To take your shoulder, chest, and back work to the next level, add the resistance exercises in chapter 9.

When Doing All the Exercises

- *Relax!* Only the muscles you are working should be tight. As you do the exercises, consciously relax your forehead and jaw. Don't furrow your brow or clench your teeth. Remember to drop your shoulders away from your ears.

- *Don't hold your breath.* When you're concentrating on a new exercise, it's easy to forget to breathe. Holding your breath deprives your exercising muscles of oxygen. It can even give you a headache. If you tend to hold your breath, then count the repetitions out loud. You can't hold your breath when you're counting.

- *Always warm up first.* Warming up gets your muscles ready for exercise by increasing their temperature and the flow of blood. A warm-up is especially important if you have been sitting all day or have been out in the cold. Before you do strengthening or resistance exercises (or aerobic activity or sports, for that matter), warm up. Gently, continuously move your arms and legs for five to ten minutes. An easy way to warm up is to walk in place. While you're walking, circle your shoulders forward and backward several times. Hunch your shoulders toward your ears, then press them away. Inhale deeply several times to expand your rib cage. Exhale deeply, too. Gently swing your arms by your sides, then from your sides to the ceiling. Slowly turn your chin toward your right shoulder, then your left, a few times.

- *Stretch the muscles you have just worked.* Stretching loosens up tight muscles, increases your range of motion, makes your movements freer and easier, increases circulation, and decreases discomfort. When done correctly, stretching feels good. Never stretch to the point of pain or burning sensation. That kind of stretching can cause microscopic tears in muscles and tendons. The resulting scar tissue will make the muscle even tighter and more inflexible. Stretching too fast or too intensely activates a protective mechanism called the stretch reflex. A nerve impulse causes the muscle to contract strongly to brace itself against injury. So the overstretched muscle actually tightens. Fast, intense

stretching does more harm than good. Stretch to the point of mild tension, then relax as you hold the stretch. Focus your attention on the muscle being stretched and try to sustain a relaxed stretch for ten to thirty seconds. The feeling of tension should subside as you relax. If it doesn't, ease up a bit.

- *Listen to your body.* Some days are more stressful and tiring than others, so you won't always be able to work at the same intensity. If you ever feel pain or discomfort in your neck, shoulders, back, hips, or knees, *stop.* You should feel your muscles work, but you should never feel discomfort in a joint. Stop, gently shake your limbs out, walk around a few minutes, then try again. If you still feel pain in your joint, then stop for the day.

2

Solving Common Posture Problems

f o u r

Get Your Head Straight

Have you ever caught your reflection in a window or mirror and noticed that your head was leading the way? A head that hangs forward is the most common posture problem. It's caused by many everyday activities, including reading books and newspapers, wearing bifocals, talking on the phone, watching television in bed, working at a computer, and leaning over a desk.

A Real Troublemaker

A head that hangs forward is not only the most widespread posture problem, but also one that causes far more problems than you might think. The reason is that a head is heavy. The average human head weighs 10 to 14 pounds, the same as a bowling ball. It's supposed to rest directly over the shoulders in the body's center of gravity. When it hangs forward even slightly it is no longer in the center of gravity, and the muscles in the neck and upper back have to work hard all the time just to hold your head up. Every inch that your head is held in front of your shoulders puts an additional fifteen

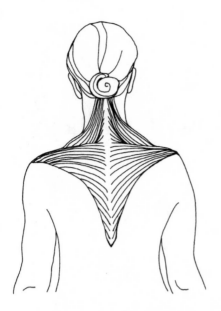

The forward-head position strains the trapezius muscle.

pounds of strain on those muscles. This starts a chain reaction.

- Most of the work is done by the upper part of the trapezius muscle (trap), a large, diamond-shaped muscle that runs from the base of the skull out to the shoulders and down to the middle back. When the head hangs forward, the upper traps are constantly under tension to hold that heavy load. Over time, they become very thick and tight. When touched, they feel like cement. This causes *stiffness and pain in the neck and upper back.*

- Because the upper trap is continually contracting, the nerves that pass between the neck bones to serve the arms and upper body get squeezed. The result can be *neck pain, numbness or tingling in the arms and hands,* or *tension headaches.* (Tension headaches, the most common type of headache, are often suffered by people whose work requires them to bend or lean forward, such as assembly-line workers, hairdressers, and dentists and dental hygienists.)

- While the upper section of the traps become overdeveloped, the middle and lower parts weaken because they don't have to work at all. The imbalance causes tremendous *discomfort in the upper and middle back.*

- The splenius cervicus, long, thin muscles that run between the skull and middle back, become stressed and strained and are often felt as *"hot spots" between the shoulder blades.*

- When your head hangs forward, unless you want to look at the floor all day, you have to lift your face by arching your neck. This puts pressure on the cartilage, disks, and joints of the neck. Over time, it increases the chance of "wear-and-tear" arthritis. The constant compression of the muscle, disks, nerves, and joints also reduces the flow of blood to the area, cutting down on the oxygen and nutrients that reach the tissues.

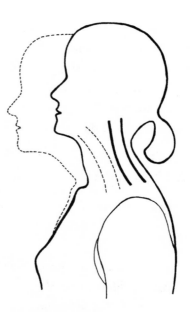

The forward-head position causes the spine to curve.

- The forward head posture is a major contributor to temporomandibular disorder (TMD), which causes *pain or clicking noises when you open and close your jaw*. TMD occurs when the hinged joint that connects the lower jawbone to the skull, and the supporting muscles, become inflamed or injured. When the head and jaw are thrust forward, as in the forward-head position, gravity pulls on the jaw and eventually the joint doesn't fit properly. TMD can be relieved by realigning the head over the shoulders and relaxing the neck muscles.

Centering Your Head Over Your Shoulders

Once you're aware of the head-forward problem, it's not difficult to correct. It just takes some attention. Lifting your rib cage, as described in *One Minute to Better Posture* (page 13), is a great start because it moves your head closer to your center of gravity. If your head has been hanging forward for years, though, that will not be enough to correct the problem. The following exercises work beautifully. All of the all-over posture improvement exercises in chapter 2 help flatten the upper back. Above all, whenever you think of it throughout the day, gently pull your head back over your shoulders.

Neck Glide

Brings the head back to the center of gravity; greatly relieves neck strain.

1. While standing or sitting, simply pull your head back over the middle of your shoulders. Think of trying to touch an imaginary wall with the back of your neck. Don't tip your head back.

2. Hold for ten seconds. Do this many times throughout the day.

Putting Your Head in Its Place

Aligns the head. Do this whenever you catch yourself with your head hanging forward; for example, when you lean over a desk, computer, or reading material.

1. Sit in a chair, but don't rest against the back. Lift your rib cage up. Pull your belly button toward your spine.

2. Stick your chin forward and then gently pull back your head and neck. Don't tip your head back or arch your neck. Instead, pretend you're trying to touch the back of your neck to an imaginary wall behind you.

3. Keeping your head high, feel the back of your neck gently stretch, and your upper back flatten.

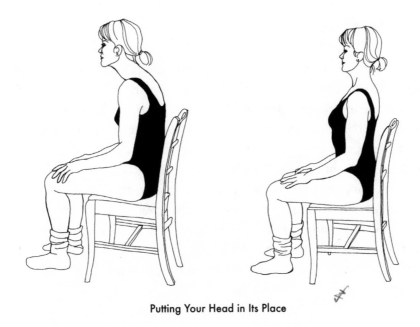

Putting Your Head in Its Place

4. Push down on your knees with your hands to help your back become as erect as possible. Hold for five seconds. Repeat several times.

Neck Straightener

Aligns the neck.

1. Lie on your back, knees bent and feet flat on the floor.

2. Put your hands under your head. Lift your head up and tuck your chin toward your chest. Then, vertebra by vertebra, *gently* place the back of your neck as close to the floor as you can *without straining*. Think of elongating your neck as much as possible.

3. When the back of your neck is as comfortably close to the floor as possible, take your hands away from your head. Hold this position for five seconds. Then relax. Repeat several times.

Neck Stretches

If your head hangs too far forward, you can bet there are extremely tight tendons and muscles in the back and on the sides of your neck. When your head hangs forward, unless you want to look at the floor all day, you have to arch your neck to lift your face. This constant arching tightens and shortens the muscles and tendons in the back of your neck and stretches the ones in the front of your neck.

Stretching exercises will reduce the muscle tension. Do the following stretches gently, adjusting to your level of flexibility. Stretch until you feel mild tension—never discomfort. Focus your attention on the area being stretched. Try to relax the muscles as you stretch them. Do not yank on your head or neck or you will defeat the purpose of the stretches. Gradually, you will gain flexibility.

Trap Stretch

Stretches the sides of the neck and the upper trapezius muscle.

1. Sit erect in a chair.

2. To stretch the right side of your neck, drop your left ear toward your left shoulder. Press your right shoulder down and reach away slightly with your right arm. Turn your face slightly to the left. Hold for ten seconds.

3. Change sides.

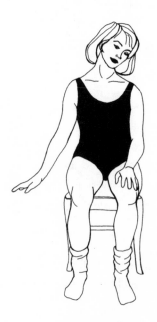

Trap Stretch

Chin-to-Chest Press

Stretches the back and sides of the neck.

1. Sit erect in a chair.

2. To stretch the left side, turn your chin toward your right shoulder. Drop your chin to your chest. Place your left hand on top of your head and gently ease your chin toward your chest (though you won't actually touch your chin to your chest). Don't force this stretch or yank on your head. Hold for ten seconds and release.

3. Repeat on the opposite side.

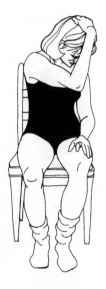

Chin-to-Chest Press

Stop Slumping

Another very common posture problem is a slumped upper back. Straightening the upper back will decrease waist measurement, increase chest measurement, restore height, provide more space for the lungs and other internal organs, and decrease those annoying, nagging aches and pains that go along with poor posture.

In a Slump

When the upper back slumps forward, it causes a lot of problems.

- The rib cage presses down on the midsection, causing the belly to protrude. The *waistline appears larger* than it really is. Standing tall eliminates the pressure on the abdominal organs, which instantly slims the waistline. You instantly lose one or more inches around the middle.

- Slumping forward exaggerates the curve in the upper part of your spine. You can *lose as much as two inches in height,* depending on how rounded your upper back is. This happens to many people as they age. If you learn at your routine doctor's checkup that you've lost one inch, your spine has curved forward that much. This is height you can and should get back, by correcting your posture.

- Slumping *decreases your chest measurement.*

- Slumping causes the *shoulders to become rounded and narrow.*

- When your chest slumps forward, your rib cage cannot expand as much as it once did, and you become a *shallow breather.* Less oxygen, and therefore less energy, reaches your body and brain.

- The downward pressure *gives your heart, liver, and stomach less room,* too.

How to Straighten Up

When the upper back slumps forward, the muscles across the middle back and between the shoulder blades are constantly stretched. They become weak and loose. The muscles in the front of the shoulders and across the chest are always contracted, so they become too short and tight. So if your chest slumps forward, you need to strengthen the muscles across the middle back and between your shoulder blades, and stretch the muscles in the front of your chest.

Wall Push-Up

Strengthens the back, chest, and arms.

Caution: Skip this exercise if you have carpal tunnel syndrome.

1. Face the wall. Bend your knees slightly and pull in your abdominals so that your pelvis is in a neutral position, not tipped forward. To make this exercise more difficult, move your feet farther away from the wall. To make it easier, move your feet closer to the wall.

2. Place your hands against the wall at shoulder level, at a distance apart of a few inches wider than your shoulders. Bend your elbows and lower your torso to the wall. Try to flatten your upper back between the shoulder blades as you lean toward the wall. Don't let the lower back sag.

3. Exhale slowly and push your body away from the wall without letting your elbows lock.

4. Repeat ten times, and gradually build to twenty-five times.

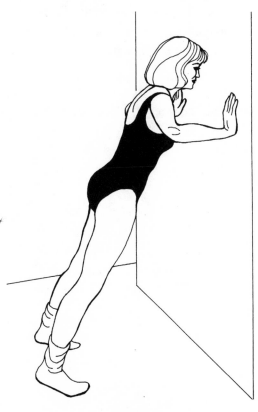

Wall Push-Up

Upper Back Arch

Strengthens muscles between shoulder blades and in the middle back; stretches the chest and the front of the shoulders.

1. Lie on your back with your knees bent and feet flat on the floor. Stretch out your arms at shoulder level with your palms facing up.

2. *Gently* press all of your spine to the floor, starting with your lower back, then mid-back, upper back, and neck. Keep your chin pulled in and your abdominal muscles tight.

3. Arch the upper back slightly. Try to lift your shoulder blades slightly off the floor. Do not let the lower back or neck arch off the floor. Hold for a slow count of five. Relax.

When you're ready to take your upper-back work to the next level, see chapter 9, "Resistance Exercises."

Straighten Your Shoulders

Many people round their shoulders over or carry one higher than the other.

Rounded Shoulders

The shoulder contains not one joint, but several. They all work whenever you move your arms.

When the shoulders are rounded, the arm bones rotate inward too much. To feel what I'm talking about, place a hand on the opposite shoulder. Rotate your arm externally, until your thumb is pointing out as if you were hitchhiking. As you rotate your arm outward, you should feel the front of your shoulder widen and flatten. You'll feel your shoulder blades retract and lie flatter. Now let the arm bone rotate inward all the way and feel what that does to your shoulder. The front of the shoulder sort of folds in on itself and the back of the shoulder becomes rounded. When your arms are rotated out slightly, or in a neutral position, your shoulders will feel wider and lie flatter. Your chest is allowed to expand, giving your lungs more room.

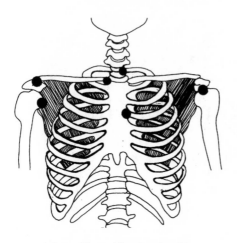

Joints affected by the shoulder

You'll breathe more deeply.

Rounded shoulders will stretch and weaken the muscles in the back of the shoulders and between the shoulder blades. The shoulder blades are higher and farther apart than they should be. The inside edges can protrude like wings instead of lying flat. On the front of the body, the shoulder muscles are constantly contracting, so they become too short and too tight.

Many people mistakenly believe that the way to straighten up is to jam their shoulders back, like a soldier—but this just causes tension in the neck. To realign all the shoulder joints, you have to rotate the arm outward and gently squeeze your shoulder blades together.

If you want to know whether your shoulders are rounded, notice where your thumbs point when you are walking along. If they point toward or rub against the outsides of your legs, your shoulders are too round. You can use the *Hitchhiker* exercise (opposite page) to adjust them easily and inconspicuously.

As you do these exercises, or any in this book for that matter, make sure you keep your head and neck pulled back and centered over your shoulders. If your head is allowed to drop forward, the chest sinks and rounded shoulders become more exaggerated. Just what you don't want.

> **Those Earrings Are Definitely Not You**
>
> Are you wearing your shoulders like earrings? Asking yourself this question several times a day will help you remember to press your shoulders down, away from your ears.

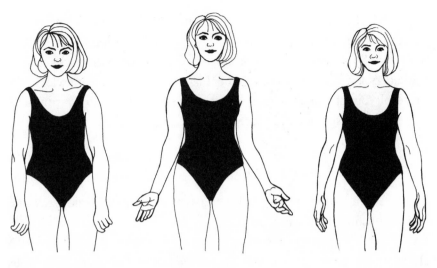

Rounded shoulders   Hitchhiker position   Neutral, correct position

Hitchhiker

Instantly unrounds the shoulders.

1. Stand with your arms hanging loosely at your sides. Lift up your rib cage. Pull your head and neck back until your head is directly over your shoulders.

2. Rotate your arms outward. Your thumbs should be pointing out as if you were hitchhiking.

3. Press both shoulders down, away from your ears.

4. Without letting your shoulders roll forward, let your arms relax. Your arm bones will roll in to a neutral position. Your palms should face your thighs and your thumbs should be pointing straight ahead. This is the anatomically correct position of the arms and hands when the shoulders are correctly aligned. If the thumbs are pointing ahead, and if your chest feels expanded and your shoulders wider, you've done it right.

While the *Hitchhiker* instantly unrounds the shoulders, as soon as you start thinking about something else, your shoulders will go back to their old ways. So the next step is to strengthen the muscles in the backs of your shoulders and between your shoulder blades and stretch the muscles in the front of your shoulders. The goal is to obtain a balance so your muscles can hold your shoulders in place without you giving them a thought.

Shoulder Unrounder

Strengthens the large muscles across the upper- and mid-back and helps unround the shoulders.

1. Sit on a chair without touching the backrest. Grab the chair seat and pull your chest up and slightly forward. Bring your head over your shoulders. Elongate your midsection. Inhale deeply. As you exhale, keep your rib cage lifted, and tighten your abdominals.

2. Breathing normally, rotate your arms until your thumbs point behind you.

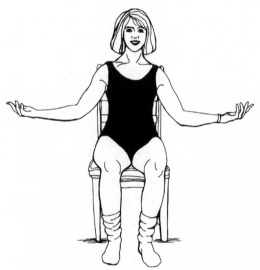

Shoulder Unrounder

Hunch your shoulders up toward your ears and then press them down.

3. Press your arms back in little movements from one to twenty times. Think of squeezing your shoulder blades toward one another each time.

4. Relax by letting your torso lean forward on your legs. Let your arms hang like deadweights.

Elbow Press

Strengthens the muscles of the middle, upper, and lower back and shoulders.

1. Sit on a chair without touching the backrest.

2. Clasp your hands behind your head. Lift your shoulders toward your ears and then press them down away from your ears. (If you feel the muscles in the back of your neck tighten while doing the rest of this exercise, you are holding your shoulders too high. Relax them and press them down. If the problem continues, skip this exercise for now and do the one above for a few weeks instead.)

3. Gently press the back of your head into your hands. You should feel the muscles along your spine tighten. Hold for five seconds.

4. Next, press your elbows back ten times. They won't move very far, but you'll feel this in the muscles between your shoulder blades.

5. Relax by letting your torso lean forward and rest on your thighs.

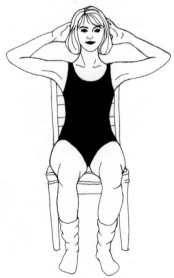

Elbow Press

Goal Post

Helps unround shoulders; strengthens the middle and upper back and abdominals; reinforces good posture.

1. Lie on your back, knees bent, feet flat on the floor. Bend your elbows and place your arms on the floor, palms up. Press your shoulders away from your ears.

2. Take a deep breath. As you exhale, tighten your abdominals and gently press your lower back toward the floor until your pelvis is in a neutral position. Then press your mid-back and then upper back into the floor until your whole spine is pressing gently into the floor. Gently ease the back of your neck as close to the floor as is comfortable. Don't force it.

3. Next, press your elbows and arms into the floor. Try to push your shoulder blades toward each other. You'll feel the muscles in the mid- and upper back tighten, especially between the shoulder blades. Hold for a slow count of ten. Then relax.

4. Slide your arms along the floor and bring your elbows toward your sides. Make sure your whole back maintains contact with the floor. Now slide your arms along the floor toward your head.

5. Repeat several times.

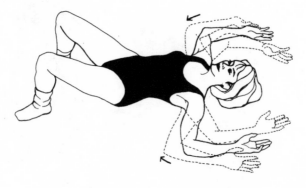

Goal Post, steps 3 through 5

Shoulder-Blade Squeeze

Strengthens the muscles between the shoulder blades and in the middle back; try this one the next time you have a tension headache!

1. Lift your rib cage. Think of pulling up with your midsection.

2. Squeeze your shoulder blades toward one another and then press them down slightly toward your waistline. Hold for a slow count of ten.

3. Repeat often.

Chest and Shoulder Stretch

Stretches the front of the shoulders and the chest.

1. Stand erect. Place your hands behind your back, one on top of the other, palms facing up.

2. Press your shoulders down, away from your ears. Lift your arms as far as is comfortable. Hold for ten seconds, then relax.

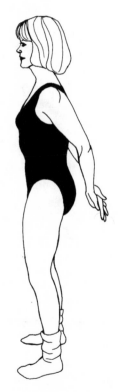

Chest and
Shoulder Stretch

Door Frame Stretch

Stretches the front of the shoulders and the chest.

1. Stand in a doorway. Stretch out your arms at shoulder level. Bend your elbows at a ninety-degree angle, so that your fingers point toward the ceiling. Face your palms onto the door frame. Tuck your pelvis under by tightening your abdominal muscles.

2. Lean your body forward until you feel a stretch in the front of your shoulders and chest. Hold for ten seconds, then relax.

3. Next, slide your elbows several inches higher. Lean your torso forward until you feel a stretch in the front of your shoulders. Hold for ten seconds, then relax.

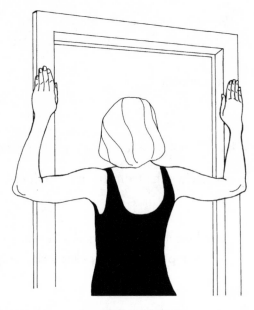

Door Frame Stretch

Uneven Shoulders

Another common shoulder problem is holding one side higher than the other. Look into a mirror to see if your shoulders are uneven. Uneven shoulders cause a lot of muscle tension. On the side that is higher, the neck muscles are tight and thick, and the muscles of the trunk are stretched. On the other side of the body, the trunk muscles shorten and contract. This muscular imbalance can eventually cause the spine to curve to one side.

To retrain your muscles, simply spend as much time as possible with your shoulders even. Here's an easy way to keep track of your shoulders throughout the day. You'll need a full-length mirror and some tape. Look in the mirror to see if one shoulder is higher than the other. Pull the higher shoulder down until you can see in the mirror that your shoulders are even. On the side of the once-higher shoulder, put a piece of tape on the place where your fingertips rest on the side of your leg or clothes. (The tape or other marker can be inconspicuous.) Throughout the day, as often as you think of it, let your fingertips find the tape on your leg or clothing. Whenever your fingertips are brushing against the tape, you'll know that your shoulders are even. To check your shoulders while you're sitting, you can pull your shoulders even and place a marker where your elbow rests against your rib cage.

The more time you spend with your shoulders correctly aligned, the more quickly your muscles will be retrained. The tape trick will help you regain your sense of balance, too. At first you'll feel off-balance, since you're used to having your shoulders slanted. Soon your body, especially your spine and neck, will come to appreciate correctly aligned shoulders and you won't need the tape as a reminder. In just a few weeks, you should see and feel results.

You also need to change habits that probably caused the problem in the first place. Try the following:

- *If you carry a purse, lighten it up, and alternate the shoulder on which you carry it.* The number-one cause of uneven shoulders in women is carrying a heavy purse on the same shoulder. To keep the strap from sliding off the shoulder, especially if a woman is round-shouldered, she has to hike up the shoulder. Day after day, year after year, this creates muscular imbalances. The muscles of the higher shoulder become tight and thick, and after a while automatically hold the shoulder in a higher position. Do you really need all that muscle tension?

- *Same goes for your briefcase or books.* If you always carry a heavy briefcase or laptop computer on one side, you'll cause stress, strain, and imbalances in the spine. At the very least, switch sides often. To carry books or notebooks to school or around campus, use a backpack instead of a bag.

- *Stand with your weight evenly on both legs.* Many people create uneven shoulders and hips because they always stand with their weight on the same leg. Try to distribute your weight evenly. If you have trouble breaking this habit, at least switch sides—shift your weight to the other leg.

- *Avoid carrying a child on your hip.* This automatically raises the hip on that side, and the shoulder comes up, too. Being a mother, I know the hip position is practical because it leaves a hand free to do things, but I urge you to use it as little as possible. Carry your child in front, close to you, with both arms. If you need to park a kid on your hip sometimes, change hips often. If you find yourself constantly carrying a baby around the house, try a baby backpack instead; it will put the weight in your center of gravity rather than on one side.

When you're ready to take your shoulder work to the next level, see chapter 9, "Resistance Exercises."

Signs of Scoliosis

Uneven shoulders and uneven hips can be a sign of scoliosis, a medical condition in which the spine is curved sidewise. The condition is often present at birth and becomes obvious during childhood or the teen years. Other times, the cause is not known. If you suspect that you or your child may have scoliosis, see your doctor. Your doctor will refer you to a physical therapist who will evaluate your condition and teach you exercises for your special needs. You may also be referred to an orthopedic surgeon, a doctor who specializes in treating disorders of bones and joints. Don't do the exercises suggested here, and don't ignore the problem. Without treatment, the problem will grow worse, causing back pain and lung problems.

seven

Lower-Back Pain

Many people experience dull, aching, or shooting pain in the lower back. Back pain can make it difficult to walk, sit, sleep, work—in fact, to do almost anything. It can make life miserable, and can even be disabling.

The number-one cause of lower-back pain is not "overdoing it" (with a sport, workout, or household chore), but simply poor posture. Most lower-back pain is caused by an exaggerated curve in the lower back, often called a "swayback." A swayback in turn is caused by weak or inflexible muscles in the abdomen, legs, buttocks, and back. You can strengthen or stretch these important muscles so they will sup-

If Your Back Aches, You're Not Alone

- Eighty-five percent of Americans will experience disabling lower-back pain at least once.

- Eighty million Americans currently have lower-back pain.

- Each year, half of all working adults have an episode of lower-back pain.

- Back injuries are the most common work injury.

- Lower-back problems cost an estimated $50 billion a year in the United States alone.

- Nonprescription pain relievers are a billion-dollar industry.

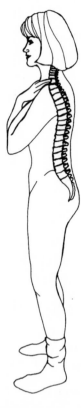

Spinal column

port the lower back and hold the pelvis in a neutral position.

If you have intense or chronic pain in your lower back, see your doctor before doing exercises, to rule out any serious conditions such as a herniated disk, scoliosis, broken bone, or osteoporosis.

The Anatomy of Your Back

The spine consists of twenty-four interlocking bones called "vertebrae." Stacked one upon another, these small bones support the weight of the body. Each vertebra contains four little joints with pain-sensitive linings. Between the vertebrae are circular pads, called "disks," composed of a soft jelly enclosed in a tough, fibrous shell. The disks separate the bones and cushion the impact of walking, running, and moving. They're the spine's shock absorbers. In a healthy back, the disks are plump and thick.

Inside this column of bones is the spinal cord, a thick bundle of nerves. Smaller nerves pass between the vertebrae and branch out to the rest of the body.

The spine has three slight curves, in the neck (the cervical curve), upper back (thoracic curve), and lower back (lumbar curve). These curves absorb shock and give the spine flexibility, while keeping the column balanced over the center of gravity. When the spine curves just the right amount, the vertebrae are stacked up properly: They glide against each other without friction. When the curves are too great, however, the spinal joints press into one another. The joint linings can become irritated and inflamed. Also, because the space between the vertebrae is narrowed when the lower back is swayed, the nerves that pass between them don't have enough room: They're pressed upon and pinched.

Too much curve in the lumbar area causes lower-back pain. If there is compression of the sciatic nerve, the person can feel anything from a dull ache to a stabbing, burning pain in the lower back, buttocks, down the leg, and even into the big toe. There can be a spot or area of pain or a line of pain down the entire leg.

Does Your Lower Back Curve Too Much?

Take this test.

- First, stand with your back and heels against a wall. Is there a tunnel between your lower back and the wall? Can you fit the palm of one hand there? Is there lots of extra room?

- Now look at yourself sideways in a mirror. Does your belly protrude? Your bottom?

- Do your knees lock back?

- Does your back ache after you've been on your feet for a while, for example after you've been to the mall or at a museum?

If you answered yes to any of the above questions, then your lower back probably curves too much.

Get Your Pelvis in Neutral

The first step in lessening the curve in your lower back is to get your pelvis in neutral. If your pelvis is in a neutral position and you lie down, your lower back will be flat or almost flat on the floor. The little bony protrusions toward the top of your pelvic bones (called the "illiac crests") should be lined up vertically with your pubic bones when you are standing or sitting, and lined up horizontally

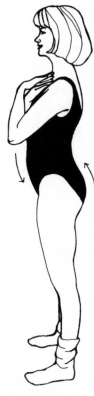
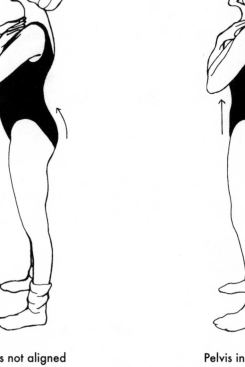

Pelvis not aligned　　　　　　　**Pelvis in neutral**

when you are lying down. Training your pelvis to be in neutral is a big step toward improving your posture and freeing yourself of lower-back discomforts.

Pelvic tilts are a great place to start. The beginner version is done in the reclining position. When you lie down, gravity assists you, making it easier to lessen the curve in your lower back. In the intermediate version, the wall helps out. If your lower-back curve has been too extreme, the soft tissue and muscles in the small of your back may have become very tight and inflexible. It'll take time to change this. If you feel discomfort while doing the pelvic tilt, stop. Try again, more gently, in a few hours.

Soon you'll be able to do a pelvic tilt without the support of the floor or wall. During the day, whenever you think of it, you'll be able to bring your pelvis into a neutral position, lessening your lower-back curve and taking the pressure off your joints, soft tissues, and nerves. Finally, you'll be able to do an advanced standing pelvic tilt; by not using your buttocks to help tilt your pelvis, you will help your abdominals work harder and become stronger.

Pelvic Tilt for Beginners

1. Lie on a bed or thick rug. Bend your knees and place your feet flat on the floor. Inhale.

2. As you exhale, squeeze your buttock muscles and tighten your abdominal muscles by pulling your belly button toward your back. Gently press your lower back into the floor until the pelvic and pubic bones line up horizontally.

3. Hold your muscles tight for a count of ten, and release. Repeat several times.

Pelvic Tilt, Intermediate Level

1. Stand with your back against a wall. Place your heels about six inches from the wall and bend your knees slightly.

2. Pull your belly button toward your spine and gently, slowly coax your lower back against the wall. Don't force anything. At first, you may have to bend your knees a lot and place your heels far away from the wall (up to twelve inches). With time, you'll be able to bend your knees less and get your feet closer to the wall. Little by little, it will happen for you.

Advanced Standing Pelvic Tilt

1. Stand with your feet hip-width apart and your knees unlocked.

2. Pull your belly button toward your back and tighten your abdominal muscles.

3. Drop your tailbone slightly. This eases the pelvis into a neutral position.

4. Hold for a slow count of five, then relax. As you become more experienced, increase the count to thirty, then for as long as you can. Try to relax your buttocks while keeping your abs tight and your hips tucked under. Don't hold your breath. Let all the other muscles in your body relax while still keeping the abdominals tight.

The next step is to train your oblique muscles, the stabilizers, to keep your pelvis in neutral while your other body parts are moving and going about their daily business. When strong, these muscles, which wrap around the sides of the body, keep your pelvis balanced and stable and provide tremendous support for the lower back.

The following exercises will help strengthen your oblique muscles. If the exercises feel easy, you're probably allowing your

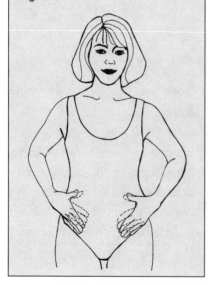

Tilt Tip

How can you know whether you're doing a standing pelvic tilt properly? Place your hands on your abdomen. Put your thumbs on the bottom of your rib cage, and your other fingers on your hipbones. As you tilt your pelvis, your fingers and thumbs should move closer together.

pelvis to move rather than keeping it perfectly still and in neutral. Have someone check you as you move your legs. The slower you exercise, the more effective you'll be, and the better you'll be able to keep your pelvis in neutral.

Ab Stabilizer, Level 1

Strengthens the oblique muscles.

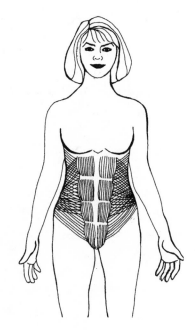

The obliques (on the sides) and rectus abdominus (middle)

1. Lie on your back, knees bent, feet flat on the floor, arms by your sides.

2. Make sure your pelvis is in neutral, then tighten your abs. Keeping the abs tight and without moving your pelvis slowly pull one knee toward your chest. Tighten the abs even more, then place that foot back on the floor *without letting the pelvis move*. If it moves even a little, the purpose of the exercise is defeated.

3. Switch knees. Do five sets.

Ab Stabilizer, Level 2

1. In the same position as above, without letting the pelvis move, first pull up one knee, then add the other.

2. Again without letting the pelvis move even slightly, place the right foot back on the floor, then the left foot. To accomplish this, you must hold your abs in extremely tight.

Ab Stabilizer, Level 3

1. Start in the same position. Keeping the knee bent at a ninety-degree angle, lift your right leg until the calf is parallel to the floor. At the same time, exhale and raise your left arm over your head. Do not let your pelvis move even a little.

2. Inhaling, bring the arm and leg back to the starting position.

3. Repeat with the opposite arm and leg.

4. See if you can do both sides three times. Gradually, build to eight times.

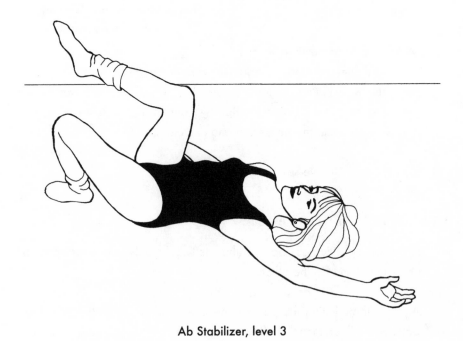

Ab Stabilizer, level 3

Standing Stabilizer

Trains the oblique muscles to keep the pelvis in neutral.

1. Stand against a wall with your pelvis in neutral and rib cage lifted.

2. Lift your arms in front of you. Without letting your pelvis or lower back move from the wall, lift your arms overhead. Lift only as far as you can and still keep your pelvis in neutral. At first, you may be surprised to find that you can't lift very far without your lower back coming away from the wall. Keep practicing. As your oblique muscles grow stronger, you'll be able to lift your arms higher while still keeping your pelvis neutral.

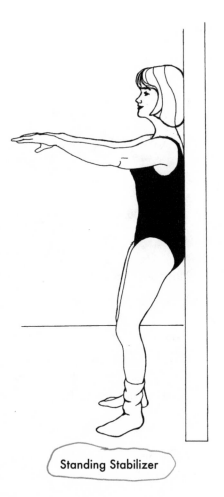

Standing Stabilizer

Relax Your Lower Back

Tight, shortened muscles in the lower back lock the pelvis into a forward tilt. The exercises described below will help relax the lower back and stretch lower-back muscles. Do them whenever you can. They feel great if you've been on your feet for a while or if you've been standing on concrete floors.

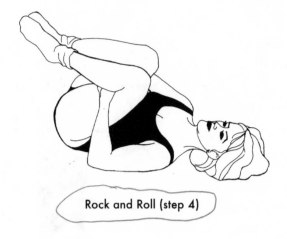

Rock and Roll (step 4)

Rock and Roll

Stretches the lower back; this feels really good, since it relieves pressure in the spinal joints and soft tissues.

1. Lie on your back and bend your knees toward your abdomen.

2. Place your hands behind your knees and gently pull your knees in toward your chest.

3. Gently rock your knees toward your chest for a few seconds.

4. Gently ease your knees toward your chest as far as they'll comfortably go. Hold for ten to twenty seconds. You should feel your lower back stretch.

5. Next, guide your knees in a circle over your chest five times in one direction and five times in the other direction.

Sink Stretch

Stretches the whole spine and feels great!

1. Hold on to the rim of a sink. Your feet should be directly under your shoulders, hip-width apart. Tuck your hips under and bend your knees a bit.

2. Let your bottom sink back slightly as if you were about to sit on the floor. Your arms should straighten but not lock. Relax your neck muscles so that your head hangs down a bit. You should feel a stretch down the length of your spine. Hold this position for ten seconds as you let your back relax.

3. Ease back to a standing position. Repeat.

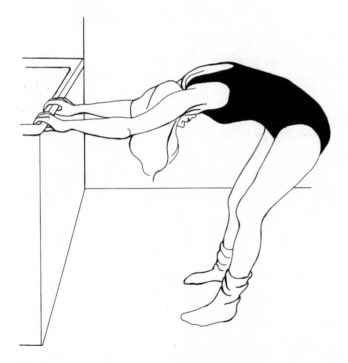

Sink Stretch

Strengthen Your Abs

There are four layers of abdominal muscles, each with fibers running in a different direction. The crisscrossing pattern shapes your midsection and supports your lower back. When the abdominal muscles are weak, the lower back sags inward, which forms a potbelly. Strong abdominals contribute greatly to the health of the total spine.

The *Pelvic Tilts* and *Ab Stabilizers* will help. Also, do the *Abdomen Tighteners* often throughout the day. These exercises will do much more for your abdominals and back than the sit-ups and ab crunches done in most exercise classes. Crunches strengthen only the rectus abdominus, the thin strip of muscle that helps you bend forward but does nothing to stabilize or support your back. The typical crunch or sit-up also pulls your neck, shoulders, and upper back into a rounded position. Have you ever had to stop doing the ab work during a class not because your abs were tired, but because your neck was killing you? The exercises are also usually done too fast—to the beat of the music. With ab work, the slower the better.

If you do crunches at a gym, here are a few tips. Don't reach forward with your arms since this encourages rounded shoulders. Pretend you have an apple or tennis ball between your chin and chest so that as you lift your head and shoulders off the floor, you won't pull your neck too far. Also, as you lift up, exhale and try to flatten your abdominals. Don't let them round out, or you'll just be wasting your time.

Abdomen Tightener 1

Strengthens the abdominal muscles to keep your lower back safe and pain-free (it even strengthens the deepest layer, which crunches can't); this exercise is totally inconspicuous and should be done as often throughout the day as you think of it.

1. Take in a deep breath. Feel your rib cage expand as your lungs fill with air.

2. As you exhale through your mouth, pull your abdominals in, as if you were trying to zip up a really tight pair of pants. Pull your belly button toward your spine and feel the bottom edge of your rib cage pull in and decrease in diameter. Hold your abdominals as tightly as you can while you slowly count to five, then relax. Gradually build up to twenty seconds. Practice holding your abdominals in tightly while still taking little breaths. Don't hold your breath.

Abdomen Tightener 2

Strengthens the abdominal muscles.

1. Inhale through your nose. Think of directing the stream of air to the area immediately below your shoulder blades. Feel the middle of your back expand backward and sideways. Your belly should not bulge forward much as you inhale.

2. Exhale through your mouth and feel your abdominals flatten and contract and the lower edge of your rib cage pull in. Hold for a slow count of ten. Then release.

3. Repeat often.

Strengthen Your Buttock Muscles

Another set of muscles that helps keep the pelvis in neutral is the buttock. When the buttock muscles are weak, they allow the pelvis to tip forward, accentuating the curve of the lower back. Again, the *Pelvic Tilts* will help. Also do the *Buttock Clencher*. It takes only takes a few seconds and can be done many times throughout the day. People who sit for many hours each day (including office workers) usually have weak, flabby butt muscles. This will help.

Buttock Clencher

Strengthens the abdominal muscles, stretches the lower back, and strengthens the buttocks.

1. Stand with your feet hip-width apart, knees slightly bent. Inhale.

2. As you exhale, pull your abdominals in and clench your buttock muscles. This brings your pelvis into a neutral position and lessens the curve in your lower back.

3. Hold for a slow count of ten, then release.

4. Repeat as many times as you can throughout the day.

Unlock Your Knees

Yet another cause of sway back is locking the knees. When a person stands with locked knees, the head of the thighbone (femur) rests against the back of the hip socket, tilting the pelvis forward and arching the lower back. Your knees are locked back if you stand with your weight on your heels. This position can also cause knee problems because your kneecaps are smashed back into your leg bones. Whenever you catch yourself standing with your knees locked back, adjust your weight so that it is spread evenly over your feet. You don't have to stand with your knees bent, but they should be in a relaxed position, not stiff and pressed backward. For more about the knees, see chapter 8.

Stretch Muscles That Can Pull the Pelvis out of Alignment

The quadriceps, hamstrings, and hip flexors are three muscle groups that, when too tight, can pull your pelvis out of neutral.

The *quadriceps* ("quads") are four muscles on the front and sides of the thigh. If the quads are very tight, they limit the range of motion in the hip joint. To accommodate the hips' decreased range of motion, the lower back has to arch and move with every step. This puts a lot of stress and strain on the lower back.

The *hamstrings* are muscles that go from the back of the lower pelvic bone to just below the back of the knee. When you take a step, they extend the thighs and bend the knees. Tight hamstrings also restrict the range of motion of the hip socket and pull on the lower back. The lower back takes the stress and strain with each step you take. To see whether your hamstrings are tight, lie on your back with your right leg bent and right foot on the floor. Extend your left leg along the floor. Keeping your left leg straight, raise it and see how far it goes while still straight. The goal is to be able to bring your leg to a ninety-degree angle while keeping the knee straight and the foot flexed. Most people have to build up to this, because their hamstrings are too tight. Below is a description of the *Hamstring Stretch*, a simple exercise that can be done at the beginning and end of the day to gain flexibility in your hamstrings quickly. You can read something while you are doing it, so that your mind is not on your hamstrings and the muscles will be allowed to relax as they stretch. You'll notice an improvement in the comfort of your lower back when your hamstrings are no longer too tight.

The *hip flexors* (iliopsoas muscles) allow you to raise a bent knee toward your chest. They are large muscles that run from the lower spine, through the abdominal cavity, to the inside of your upper thigh. When they are too tight, they pull your lower back into an arch. Tight hip flexors are very common. Ironically, athletic activity is often a contributing factor.

The following stretches will help your hip joints move more easily and freely, increasing the comfort of your lower back. Always stretch only until you feel mild tension, never burning or discomfort.

Reclining Quad and Flexor Stretch

Stretches the quadriceps and hip flexors.

1. Lie on your right side and rest the side of your head in the palm of your hand or on your right arm, whichever is most comfortable.

2. Bend your left leg and grab the left ankle with your left hand. Ease the thigh back as far as is comfortable. Keep the left thigh parallel to the floor.

3. Hold for ten seconds and release. Change sides.

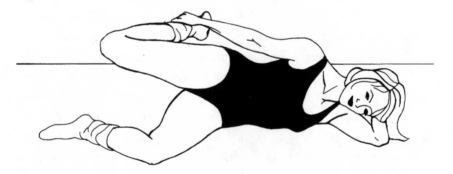

Reclining Quad and Flexor Stretch

Standing Quad and Flexor Stretch

Stretches the quadriceps and hip flexors.

1. Place your left hand on a wall or on the back of a chair for balance. Bend your right knee and raise your foot behind you. Grab your right ankle with your right hand and ease your right foot as close to your buttocks as is comfortable. Your knees should be side by side, and your trunk vertical (not leaning forward or back). Make sure the standing leg is slightly bent, not locked. You'll feel a stretch up the front of your leg and in the front of your hip. To increase the stretch, press your hips forward slightly.

2. Hold for ten seconds. Over time, build up to twenty seconds. Release and change legs. If one leg is tighter than the other, spend more time on it.

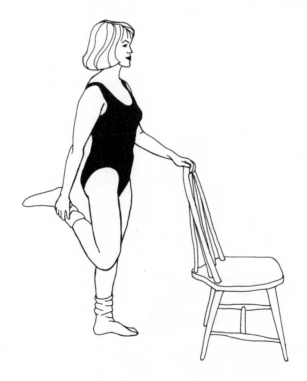

Standing Quad and Flexor Stretch

Hamstring Stretch

Increases flexibility in the hamstrings.

1. Grab a book or magazine before you start. Place a thick rug or mat by a doorway.

2. Lie on your back with your bottom about twelve inches away from the doorjamb. Put one leg through the opening of the door. Bend that leg, and put the foot flat on the floor. Place the other leg up the side of the door. Adjust your position closer to the wall or farther away until you feel a good, comfortable stretch down the back of the raised leg. If you feel this more behind your knees than anywhere else, the stretch is too intense and you should slide your bottom farther from the wall. As you become more flexible, bring your buttocks closer and closer to the wall. Soon

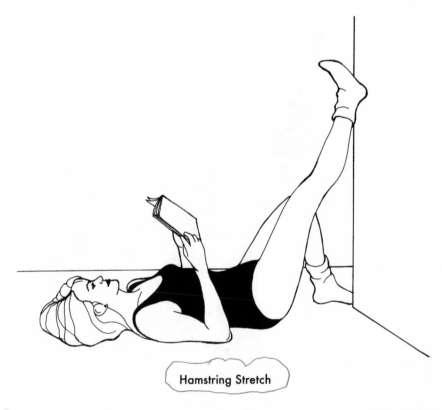

Hamstring Stretch

you'll be able to get your bottom right against the wall with your leg straight up.

3. Hold this position while you read for several minutes.

4. Switch legs and repeat. Many people find that one leg is tighter than the other. Spend more time stretching the tighter leg.

Your Knees and Feet

Correct alignment begins at your base; that is, your knees, ankles, and feet. They have to support the weight of your entire body. If they aren't aligned properly, you can get sore knees, aching ankles, bunions, and weak arches.

If you have painful knees because of an injury or surgery, ask your doctor to refer you to a physical therapist to evaluate your problem and prescribe specific exercises.

Your Knees

Have you taken a good look at your knees lately? Take off your shoes and socks and roll up your pants, then turn sideways and look in a mirror. First, are your knees stiff and locked back? When you stand, your knees should be in an easy, neutral position, straight or slightly bent. Standing with your knees locked back and your weight on your heels jams the kneecap into the leg bones, contributes to a sway back, and weakens the quadriceps (the muscles on the front of your thighs) and abdominals (because they're constantly stretched).

To feel the effects of locked knees, stand with your knees locked back. Lean forward slightly and place your hands on the front of your thighs. You'll find that the quads are loose and slack. Feel your kneecaps. Notice how they can jiggle around. Now unlock your knees and bend them slightly. Put hands on your quads and you'll find that they are firmer and that your kneecaps are held firmly in place. When you stand with your knees locked, the front thigh muscles don't have to work as much and can become weaker and weaker. Every time you catch yourself with your knees locked back, release them to an easy position.

Look in the mirror again. Do your kneecaps turn inward toward each other? Do they pull to the outside of the leg? When your knees are aligned properly, the kneecaps point straight ahead. If the kneecaps roll in toward one another, you probably need to strengthen the outside of your thighs and stretch the inside of your thighs. If the kneecaps pull to the outside of the leg, then the outside of your thighs may be too tight. You need to stretch the outside of your thigh and strengthen the inside.

Bend your knees simultaneously and look down between them. Do they track directly over your feet or do they come to the inside? You should see the big toes of each foot when you look down in this position. If you can't, then the knees are misaligned and every time you bend your knees you are wearing away the joint linings, little by little. Do the following simple movement whenever you have a few spare moments.

Knee Straightener

Realigns knees to ankles.

1. Stand with your feet hip-width apart. Make sure your feet are pointing straight ahead.

2. Press your big toes into the floor.

3. Place your hands on the insides of your thighs.

4. Slowly bend your knees while gently pressing your thighs out with your hands, so the knees go directly over the feet. Keep the big toes pressed into the floor as you do this.

5. Bend and straighten your knees ten to twenty times. Note: If this feels uncomfortable, don't bend as far. If it is still uncomfortable, you need to see a physical therapist.

Your Feet

The foot contains twenty-six bones and numerous muscles. Take off your socks and shoes and look at your ankles. Do they roll in? Are your arches flat? Do you have bunions or calluses? Are your toes straight or bent? Does the big toe pull inward toward the other toes? These problems are all related to posture.

Most foot problems are caused by wearing shoes with heels that are too high and toe boxes that are too narrow. Wearing high heels alters the position of every weight-bearing joint in your body. Heels higher than one inch increase a swayback, which leads to lower-back discomfort. The foot slides to the front of the shoe, which puts way too much pressure on the ball of the foot and all the toes. High heels shorten the Achilles tendon on the back of the calf and foot and stretch and weaken the muscles on the front of the ankle, which can lead to shinsplints. Heels on shoes also get in the way of your natural stride, which is to place the heel down first, then roll through the ball of the foot.

The lower the heel, the better. Even a one-inch heel causes a twelve-degree tilt in the ankle joint, which in turn causes all the other joints to adjust so you don't topple over. If a building were tilted twelve degrees, the doors and windows wouldn't work properly. Of course, a building can't make adjustments like a human body can. Our bodies adjust, but we eventually pay for it with stiff, aching joints and painful feet. The heel of your foot should be as close to the ground as possible.

Wearing footwear with narrow or pointed toe boxes pushes the big toe toward the other toes. When the big toe has been pushed out of alignment for years, the muscular arch under the inside of your foot flattens and weakens. Flat arches cause problems not only for your feet, but also for your ankles, knees, hips, and even back, since all parts are connected and depend on one another to work correctly and efficiently.

The soles of your shoes should be flexible, both lengthwise and from side to side. With each step, the human foot is supposed to roll from the heel to sole to toe. If shoes are inflexible, the natural roll is impossible, so the muscles, tendons, and joints of the feet can't work properly. This can lead to fallen arches and ankle problems.

Shoes with built-in arch supports work well if they actually fit your foot correctly. If not, they'll just rub against your foot and create friction. If you have high arches, flat feet, or painful feet, make an appointment with a podiatrist for a custom insole. The podiatrist will make a mold of the bottom of your foot and create an insole to fit your foot exactly.

The most important way to help your feet is to get rid of any shoes that are causing problems and buy yourself some slightly longer, broad-toed, flat, flexible shoes. Yes, they can still look good, and your feet will love them.

Tight nylons and socks can squash all of the toes together and bend them under, causing hammertoes. After you put on socks or stockings, stretch the toe area to the side and wiggle your toes inside. This will create room for the toes to be straight.

You can save your joints a lot of wear and tear by putting cushioned insoles into your shoes to absorb the impact of walking, particularly on asphalt and cement. A good choice is a sorbothane insole, a thin, flat (no built-in arches), rubbery insole that can be trimmed with scissors to fit your shoes. Look for them in sporting goods stores.

If you have weak or fallen arches, the following exercises will really help. In addition, do the anytime/anywhere exercise *Buttock*

Clencher (chapter 7) often throughout the day. Pinching the butt muscles together not only decreases a sway back, but lifts the arches of the foot. The contracting butt muscles would slightly rotate the thighbone outward if friction between the soles of your feet and the floor weren't preventing your feet from rotating outward. The rotary force is transmitted to your feet and the arches lift. Give it a try. Stand tall with your feet hip-width apart and toes pointing straight ahead. Clench your butt—think of pinching the muscles together. Feel your lower back stretch and your arches pull up.

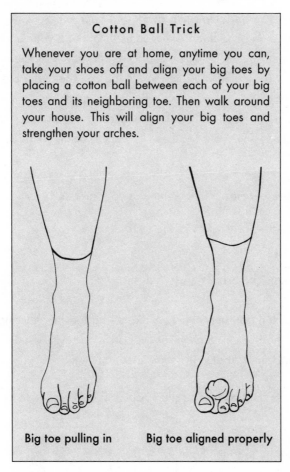

Cotton Ball Trick

Whenever you are at home, anytime you can, take your shoes off and align your big toes by placing a cotton ball between each of your big toes and its neighboring toe. Then walk around your house. This will align your big toes and strengthen your arches.

Big toe pulling in   Big toe aligned properly

Lining Up Your Big Toes

Realigns big toes that are pointing in; strengthens the arch of the foot.

1. To ease your big toes into the proper alignment with the rest of your foot, place a cotton ball between each big toe and the neighboring toe. (If you find that the cotton balls fall out during this exercise, you can tape them in place.) The cotton ball should be thick enough to straighten the big toe.

2. Stand with your feet hip-width apart and your knees slightly bent. Press your big toes into the floor. At the same time, bend your knees and gently press them outward; when you look between your bent knees, you should be able to see your big toes. If you can't see your big toes, place your hands on the insides of your thighs and gently press your knees outward. Hold this position for a few seconds and then release. When you press the knees out, your big toes will want to come off the floor. Don't let them.

3. Repeat several times. You'll feel this in your arches.

Golden Arches

Strengthens the arches and ankles.

1. Place a cotton ball between your big toe and its neighboring toe. Holding on to the back of a chair for support, stand with your feet hip-width apart, head pulled back, rib cage lifted, abs tight.

2. Roll onto the balls of your feet, keeping your ankles straight. Don't let them bow out.

3. Lower your heels to the floor.

4. Repeat ten times. Gradually work your way up to fifty times.

High-Heel Blues

Stretches the Achilles tendons and calf muscles.

1. Stand with the balls of your feet on a book or the bottom stair of a staircase. Let your heels hang lower than the toes until you feel a good stretch in the back of your ankles.

2. Hold for twenty seconds. Repeat several times throughout the day.

Banishing a Bunion

A bunion is excessive bone growth at the base of the big toe. It causes inflammation and irritation. Most bunions are caused by wearing shoes with narrow toe boxes that push the big toe toward the other toes. In turn, the joint at the base of the big toe is forced outward so it continually rubs against the side of the shoe, and a bunion forms there. If you have bunions, do the exercises noted in this chapter to help realign the big toe and strengthen your arches. Buy shoes with very wide toe boxes to take away the constant rubbing. With patience, strengthening exercises, and wide enough shoes, the bunion should become smaller and smaller. If the bunion is large or painful or recurs, see a doctor who specializes in foot problems. Unless treated, the problem will grow worse.

Resistance Exercises

The exercises in this section require exercise tubes or bands to help you take your posture-strengthening program a step further. The tube or band provides dynamic resistance to help you gain muscular strength and endurance quickly and easily. These exercises focus on the shoulders, mid, and upper back—the places people are most likely to have posture problems.

In my workshops, people of all ages and all levels of strength have really enjoyed using the resistance bands and have found them an efficient way to exercise. Not only do the bands help you improve your posture by strengthening your back and shoulders, but they'll make your arms strong—an excellent side benefit. When first starting out, do one or two repetitions of each exercise and see how it feels. Start slowly and gradually build strength.

Exercise tubes are made of rubber. You can buy them in stores that sell fitness equipment and other sporting goods. Exercise bands, which are flat and made of latex, are often used in physical therapy. You can order them from Fitness Wholesale (1-800-537-5512) or Spri Products (1-800-222-7774). Both products come in three thicknesses, for light, medium, and heavy resistance. I suggest you start with the lightest resistance level and work your way up.

Working with a Tube or Band

- Always warm up first for five to ten minutes. Gently move your arms and legs by walking, riding an exercise bike, or doing another activity.

- Stretch after each exercise to release tension, improve circulation, and increase flexibility in the muscle group that was just worked. Do one of the relaxation movements described at the end of this section after each set.

- Use slow, controlled movements. Never hyperextend or lock the joints. Breathe evenly the whole time. Don't hold your breath.

- Make sure your shoulders don't creep up toward your ears. Keep them relaxed and pressed down.

- Body alignment is extremely important. Keep your rib cage lifted, but not bowed, your shoulders relaxed and squared, your abdominals tight and pulled in toward your spine. Keep your head over your shoulders. It is really easy to let your head drop forward. Don't let it.

- The exercises can be performed while sitting in a chair or standing, whichever is more comfortable for you.

- There are three ways you can hold the tube or band. First, you can place it between your thumb and index finger and fold all four fingers over the ends. Second, you can wrap the band around your hand once or twice (this position provides a firm hold but can diminish circulation to your hands; be sure to release the band after each set). Or, you can place an end of the band or tube in the palm of each hand and wrap your fingers over it. Choose the position that is most comfortable for you.

- Don't bend your wrists while doing the exercises. Keep your hands straight to the wrists and don't let them be pulled out of alignment.

- You can make the exercises easier by sliding your hands further away from one another on the band. You can make them more difficult by placing your hands closer together. When you begin, test each exercise with your hands far apart on the band. See how it feels, then adjust your hands according to your level of strength.

- You should check with your doctor before doing resistance exercises if you have a history of high blood pressure; shoulder injury, dislocation, or crepitus (grinding, snapping); or carpal tunnel syndrome.

Strengtheners

Rhomboid Squeeze

Helps flatten the upper back.

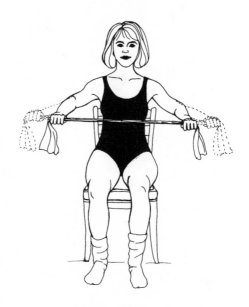

Rhomboid Squeeze

1. Lift your rib cage up and bring your head directly over your shoulders. Relax your shoulders and tighten your abdominals.

2. Grab the band so that your hands are about shoulder-width apart. Bring the band in front of you, just below chest level. Your arms should be extended but slightly bent. Pull your elbows back. Squeeze your shoulder blades. Don't let your chest bow forward as your elbows come back. Hold the position for a count of three and slowly release to the starting position.

3. Build to twelve repetitions. Keep your shoulders pressed down, away from your ears, so the muscles at the sides of your neck don't tighten.

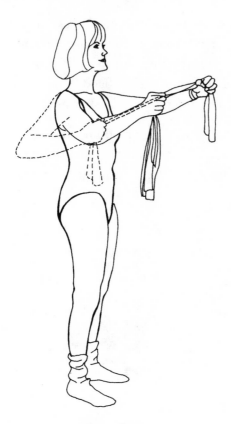

Bow and Arrow

Bow and Arrow

Strengthens shoulders and mid- and upper back.

Note: To increase this exercise's effectiveness, do a few reps, then lower the straight arm several inches and do a few more reps. Keep lowering the arm a few inches at a time until it is chest level. This changes the angle of resistance and works many muscles.

1. Lift your rib cage up and align your head over your shoulders. Press your shoulders down and tighten your abs.

2. Grab the band with your left hand and extend that arm in front of your body slightly above chest level, keeping the elbows slightly bent.

3. Grab the other end of the band with your right hand. Pull your right elbow back and down in one smooth motion. Hold for a few seconds and release. Build up to twelve repetitions. Change arms.

Shoulder Raises

Strengthens shoulders and corrects rounded shoulders.

1. Stand with your feet hip-width apart, knees slightly bent, abdominals pulled in, rib cage lifted, head aligned.

2. With your arms hanging by your sides, grab the band with your hands. Gently pull your shoulder blades toward each other.

3. Holding the band steady with your right hand, raise your left arm *without letting your shoulder blades or torso move*. At first, raise your arm about 45 degrees, then slowly release. As you become stronger, you can raise your arm to just below shoulder level. Build up to twelve repetitions. Change arms.

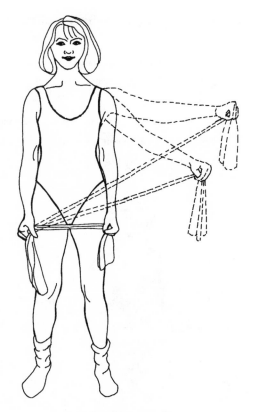

Shoulder Raises

Shoulder Strengthener

Strengthens the muscle that rotates the shoulder.

Note: Use a band with very light resistance for this exercise.

1. Lift your rib cage up, press your shoulders away from your ears, and tighten your abdominals. Hold the band with your left hand.

2. Bring your elbows to your sides and extend your forearms straight out in front. Gently pull your shoulder blades toward each other, then *don't let them move* during the exercise.

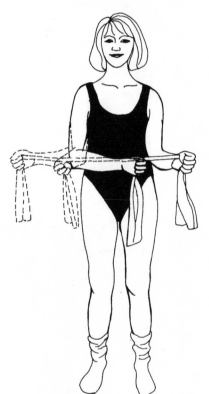

3. Bring your right forearm across your midsection and grab hold of the band about six inches from the left hand.

4. Keeping your elbows glued to your sides, pull your right forearm away from your midsection until it is by your side. For some this will be enough of an exercise. Others may be able to bring the right arm even further away from the midsection.

5. Build to twelve repetitions. Change sides.

Shoulder Strengthener

Horizontal Shoulder Press

Strengthens the shoulders and the backs of the arms.

1. Grip the band with your right hand and place that hand on your chest.

2. With the left hand, grab the band six inches away from the other hand.

3. Raise your left elbow a few inches below shoulder level.

4. Extend your forearm until the whole arm is straight. Don't let your shoulders creep up. Keep them pressed down.

5. Hold the position for three seconds and slowly release.

6. Build up to twelve reps. Then change arms.

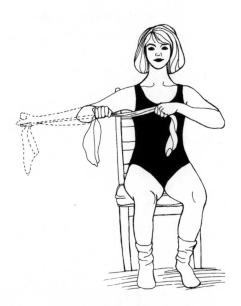

Horizontal Shoulder Press

Stretches

Between each set of resistance exercises, do the relaxation movement that will stretch the muscle group you just worked. Do these movements without the exercise band or tube.

Shoulder Stretch

Relaxes the shoulder and middle back.

1. Bring your right arm across the front of your chest.

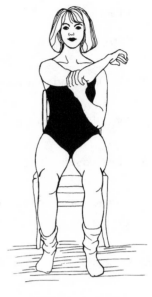

Shoulder Stretch

2. Grab your right elbow with your left hand and gently pull your elbow across your chest toward the opposite shoulder. Hold for ten to twenty seconds.

3. Change arms.

Rhomboid Release

Relaxes the muscles between your shoulder blades.

1. Interlace your fingers, palms out.

2. Stretch your arms out in front of your chest. Round your upper back slightly and feel your shoulder blades ease away from one another. Hold for ten seconds.

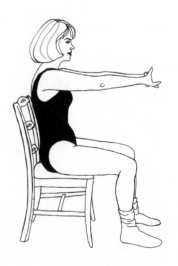

Rhomboid Release

3

Good Posture All Day Long

t e n

Sitting Down on the Job

W e're a nation of professional sitters. If you are an office worker, computer operator, or student, you probably spend a good part of your day sitting. Sitting for a long time is a major cause of back discomfort: it puts continuous pressure on the muscles and disks of the lower back. You may think that your back muscles get a rest when you sit. Actually, they're working very hard to hold you upright. *Sitting puts 40 percent more pressure on the lower back than standing does.*

Sitting is particularly hard on the lower back, especially if you sit with your lower back rounded over (called "forward flexion"). Make sure you sit with your pelvis in neutral: The top of the pelvic bones (illiac crests) should line up with the pubic bones (see page 59). This is much less stressful for your lower back. Leaning over a desk and looking up and down from a keyboard to a computer screen puts pressure on the neck and upper back, too. By stopping the slouch, supporting your back properly, and avoiding the head-forward position, you will be able to work more comfortably and productively.

Replacing or modifying your office furniture is a good start. Fortunately, more manufacturers are producing furniture and accessories with good posture in mind. A new industry has popped up: ergonomic furniture. Ergonomics is the study of equipment design to help reduce the user's fatigue and discomfort, and to increase productivity. In theory, this is great. However, marketing people also use the word "ergonomic" more loosely, to mean comfortable, easy to use, or efficient. Keep in mind that a piece of furniture is ergonomically correct *for you* only if it fits your particular body.

In any case, furniture alone can't help your posture. You also have to become more aware of how you sit and you need to take little breaks during the day.

Setting Up a Computer Workstation

If you work at a computer, try to make as many of the following adjustments to your desk and chair as possible. They will take away most of the causes of back and neck discomfort.

- Make sure your work surface is at elbow level. If it's too low, place blocks under the legs of the desk. If it's too high, raise your chair seat and use a footrest.

- The top of the computer screen should be at eye level. This will let your eyes fall comfortably on the screen. Your head will be balanced over your spine, not tilted forward or backward. If your screen is too low, put it on a computer base or on books. If your screen is too high, lower it.

- Your torso should be an arm's length from the computer screen.

- The keyboard should be slightly angled toward you, not flat. Many keyboards have a built-in "prop" at the back. If yours doesn't, place a thin book or magazine under the back end.

- At the keyboard, your wrist should be straight, not flexed down or up (see the section about carpal tunnel syndrome, below).

- The ideal computer chair has adjustable armrests that support your arms at elbow level. Both the width and height of the rests should be adjustable. Armrests relieve a quarter of the load on the lower back and take the burden of supporting the arms off the back, which allows the upper back muscles to relax more. An adjustable width is important for women because most office chairs are built to accommodate the average man; if the

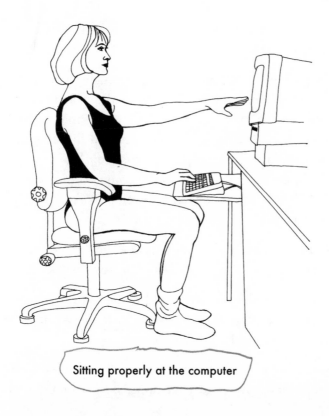

Sitting properly at the computer

armrests are too wide, you won't be able to use them for support.

- The ideal chair will support the width and length of your back. At the very least, the chair back should reach to your shoulder blades. The chair back should be either perfectly straight or at an incline of no more than ten percent.

- Your buttocks and the middle of your back should make contact with the backrest.

- The chair seat should be padded with rounded edges, and slightly tilted. The back of the seat should be slightly lower than the front, so that the buttocks can be placed against the back of the chair and the knees can be slightly higher than the hips.

- Your knees should extend no more than a few inches from the edge of the seat.

- The chair seat should be long enough to support the whole length of your thighs. That way, the weight of your body is evenly distributed over your buttocks and the full length of your thighs. People with long legs find that most seats are too narrow for them; they often cross their legs to support at least the upper leg fully; but a cross-legged position causes muscular imbalances in the hips and lower back, so it's much better to find a chair that's right for you.

- Your feet should rest flat on the floor. Adjust the height of the seat or get a footrest. A telephone book works in a pinch.

- Your chair should swivel and be on casters so you can adjust your reach and line of vision without twisting, bending, or leaning forward.

- Use a copy holder to put your work at eye level, so your head won't hang over and your upper back won't round over. You want to tilt the angle of your work—not the angle of your head on your neck.

Avoiding Carpal Tunnel Syndrome

Flexing your wrists while doing repetitive hand and finger movements, such as typing or working a cash register, places you at higher risk for developing carpal tunnel syndrome: numbness, tingling, burning, or pain in the middle and index fingers and thumb (and sometimes all the fingers). Eventually, your hand grip may weaken. Carpal tunnel syndrome is increasingly common among office workers. You can reduce your risk by modifying your workstation and changing the way you use your hands.

Hand and finger movements repeated over and over for a long time, especially when the wrists are lower than the hand, cause inflammation around the median nerve, which runs through a narrow tunnel of bone and ligament in the middle of the wrist. Since bones and ligaments have no give, this puts pressure on the nerve and causes the symptoms.

If you have any of the above-mentioned symptoms, see your doctor for diagnosis and treatment. Early intervention can help prevent and minimize symptoms. Stop the problem before it becomes severe and permanently damages your wrist.

> ### Retrofitting a Chair
>
> If you can't buy a new chair, try these inexpensive ways to adjust the seat height, back support, and armrests.
>
> • If the seat is too low and the armrests are too high, place a cushion on the seat to raise your body. Use a telephone book or box as a stool for your feet.
>
> • If the chair depth was made for a person with longer legs, place a cushion between the chair back and your body.
>
> • If you don't have armrests, try placing a box on your lap and resting your elbows on it.
>
> • To prevent your lower back from slouching backward, place a small Lumbar pillow behind you to remind you to sit with your pelvis in neutral.

If you work at a keyboard, and especially if it causes you discomfort, also try to make the following changes at work:

- When using your keyboard, keep your wrists straight—neither flexed downward nor extended upward. Bending the wrist narrows the tunnel through which the median nerve passes, so it worsens the problem.

- Rest your hands periodically throughout the day.

- If you can, rotate work activities so you don't spend hours at a time at the keyboard.

- Exercises that strengthen the hand and arm muscles may help. When these muscles are weak, there's a tendency to compensate with poor wrist position.

- If you are experiencing the symptoms of carpal tunnel syndrome, a physical therapist can design splints for you to wear while you work, which protect your wrists and keep them in a neutral position. The splints will be specific to the kind of work that you do. You may want to wear a wrist splint at night. It will keep your wrist in a neutral position so symptoms don't wake you. It may also reduce your symptoms during the daytime.

For a Desk Without a Computer

The same features of a good chair apply if you work at a desk without a computer. The top of the desk should be at elbow level.

Angling the surface of your workstation prevents you from having to lean over your work. Constantly leaning the head forward over a desk causes so much back and neck misery! Office-supply stores sell inexpensive drafting boards that can be placed on top of a desk. You can also prop up a clipboard. Adjust the surface so you are looking straight ahead rather than down. A raised work surface will enable you to sit and work with your back and head straight and balanced. You could also tilt the desk surface toward you by putting books or boards under the back legs of the desk. Propping up your work surface, however you can, will allow you to work with your head directly over your spine.

The way you talk on the phone can cause posture problems, too. Don't clench your phone receiver between your ear and shoulder. If you need to keep your hands free, get a wireless headset.

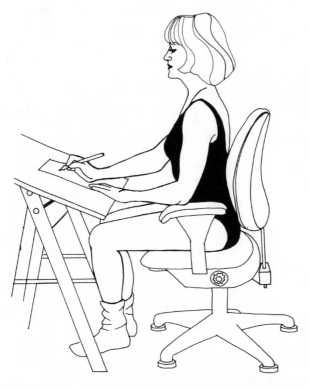

Tilting a desk surface

Exercises at Work

You can do these exercises right at your desk. They'll relieve stress in both your body and mind. Work them in throughout the day. Also, take a one-minute break to stand up and stretch once an hour.

Stretch and Grow

Elongates the spine.

1. Lift up from your midsection. Think of separating your ribs from your hipbones. Pull your abs in snugly.

2. Breathing normally, practice walking with your midsection elongated.

Exhale and Relax

Relaxes muscles whenever you feel tense.

1. Inhale through your nose. Think of inhaling into the tight muscle, whether it is your upper back or sides of neck or lower back.

2. When you exhale, consciously relax the tight muscle. Exhale all of the tension.

3. Repeat several times.

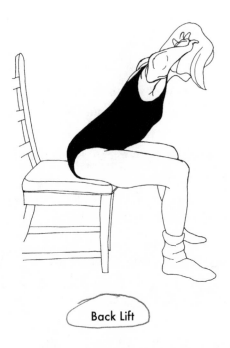

Back Lift

Back Lift

Strengthens the muscles of the lower back.

1. Sit on the edge of a chair. Clasp your hands behind your head.

2. Bend forward as far as you comfortably can. Then slowly lift your head and torso until your back and neck are at a forty-five-degree angle to the floor. As you lift, squeeze your shoulder blades together.

3. Repeat eight times.

Take a Break

Total-body stretch.

1. Raise your shoulders toward your ears and then press them down as far as possible. Hold for five to ten seconds. Repeat twice.

2. Circle your shoulders, five times in one direction, five times in the other.

3. Squeeze your shoulder blades together, then press them down. Hold for a count of five and relax. Repeat three times.

4. Clasp your hands behind your head. Relax and drop the shoulders. Press your elbows back, squeezing your shoulder blades together. Hold for five seconds, then relax. Repeat three times.

5. Clasp your hands behind your waist. Slowly lift the clasped hands away from your body. Feel your chest muscles stretch and your shoulder blades pull toward one another. Hold for five seconds and relax. Repeat three times.

6. Take a deep breath and feel your rib cage expand. As you exhale, tighten your abdominals as much as possible. Pull them in as if you were trying to zip up a really tight pair of pants. Hold the muscles tight for a slow count of five, then relax. Repeat several times.

7. Spend a few seconds doing the *Shoulder Unrounder* (page 50).

eleven

Behind the Wheel

We all spend a lot of time coming and going in our cars. Most of the time, we're slumped over the wheel. The next time you're waiting for a red light, look into the nearby cars. The drivers' heads will probably be hanging forward, their upper backs rounded over. This position not only contributes to poor posture in general, but is also tiring during a long drive. Good posture can help a driver stay comfortable and alert.

Adjusting Your Car Seat

You can adjust your seat so it will help keep your body properly aligned while you drive. All these little adjustments will make a big difference in your posture and comfort.

1. Move the seat close enough to the pedals and steering wheel that your knees are bent and your bottom rests against the back of seat. If the seat is too far away from the pedals, you will not be able to sit with your pelvis in neutral or with your bottom against

the seat back. However, for air-bag safety, you should be no closer to the steering wheel than twelve inches.

2. You want to be able to rest against the back of the seat and still sit up straight. Bring your seat to its straightest position. Ideally, it should incline no more than ten degrees.

3. Adjust the headrest so that you can sit with the back of your head resting against it. This position puts your head directly over your spine and allows your neck muscles to relax while you drive. It is also safer in case you are rear-ended; when the headrest sits at neck level, your head can snap back over it in a collision. If your car's headrest tilts too far back, make it thicker by attaching a rolled-up towel with rubber bands.

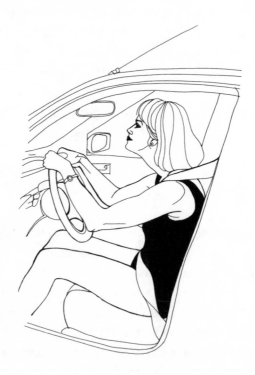

Look familiar?

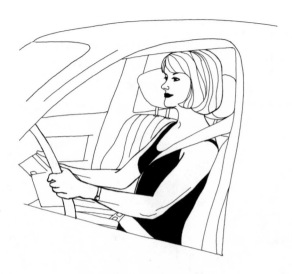

Good driving position

4. In driver education classes we all learned to hold the steering wheel in the ten o'clock and two o'clock positions. This encourages the driver to round the shoulders and raise the shoulders and arms, causing unnecessary tension in the shoulder and neck muscles. Instead, get a lower grip on the steering wheel, at nine o'clock and three o'clock. In this position, the upper arms hang more vertically and the shoulders are less hunched, which allows the neck muscles to relax, greatly reducing discomfort and fatigue.

Car Exercises

All those trips in your car are opportunities to build some posture work into your daily routine. Talk about turning things around—your car can help your posture instead of harming it!

The following exercises can be done *while you're stopped at red lights*. (Don't try to do them while you're driving along.) They will help strengthen the mid- and upper back and abdominals. If you're on a long trip, they'll refresh you, too—do them at the rest area or when you stop for lunch. If you're a passenger, you can exercise while you're rolling along.

- Lift up your rib cage and press the back of your head against the headrest. Stay lifted that way while you drive.

- Press the back of your shoulders into the seat as if you were trying to bring your shoulder blades closer together. Hold for ten seconds, then relax. Repeat several times.

- Tighten your abdominals. Take a deep breath. As you exhale, pull your belly button toward your spine and hold for ten seconds. See if you can feel the bottom of your rib cage pull in. Don't hold your breath. You need to learn how to hold your abdominals in tightly and still breathe, even if they are little breaths. Gradually build up to holding the abdominals for thirty seconds. Then see if you can hold them in until one minute clicks by on your car clock. See if you can hold them in until one song finishes on the radio. As soon as your mind wanders, your abs will probably relax, but every second you hold them in helps.

- Lengthen your midsection. Pretend your spine is growing longer. Think of pulling your rib cage away from your hip-bones. Pull your abdominals in snugly. See how long you can maintain this elongation at red lights.

- Hug yourself by placing your hands on the opposite shoulders. While keeping your hands on your shoulders, press your elbows forward and round your upper back to stretch the muscles between your shoulder blades.

t w e l v e

Sleeping

If you've ever met the dawn feeling like you were run over by a truck, you know that posture matters when you're sleeping, too. Certain sleeping positions can intensify a swayback or give you a pain in the neck. Considering that you spend about a third of your life sleeping, your position can make a big difference in your overall posture as well as the comfort of your nights and mornings.

Most people who get an aching back while sleeping assume that the problem is their mattress. Unless the mattress is lumpy or sags one way or the other, it doesn't matter as much as the position in which you sleep. The most important thing is to keep your head level with your spine. Often the solution is a few well-placed pillows. Proper support of the body can take a lot of stress off the joints of the spine.

Sleeping on Your Side

The side is a good sleeping position, but it creates the widest gap between your neck and the mattress. Side sleepers need a firm pillow

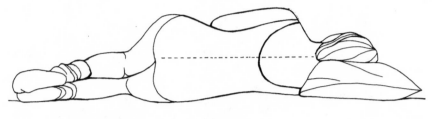

Straight spine

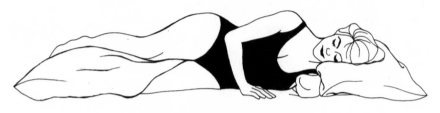

Placing a pillow between your legs

that provides lots of support for the neck. Foam pillows give more support than cushy down ones. The pillow or pillows should be as wide as the distance from your ear to the end of your shoulder. If the pillows aren't high enough, your head will tilt down toward the mattress and your shoulder will really roll under—not good if you already tend to have rounded shoulders. Your pillow has to be wide enough to support your head and keep it in neutral (that is, level with your spine), but not so wide that it tilts your head toward the ceiling. Ask your significant other or a friend to check your sleeping position.

When you lie on your side with your knees stacked on top of one another, the weight of the top thigh pulls on the joints in the lower spine and the hip socket. You can take the pressure off by placing a regular-size bed pillow between your knees and lower legs. You'll find this extremely comfortable, especially if you have lower back or hip discomfort. If you roll to your other side during the night, your body will soon learn to take the pillow along.

Sleeping on Your Back

Back sleepers should put a pillow or rolled-up beach towel under their lower legs. When the lower legs are elevated, the lower back is in a more stretched position, which takes pressure off the spinal joints. Because of the way the leg bone fits into the hip socket, when you lie down with your legs straight out, the top of the pelvis tilts forward, creating a big gap between the lower back and mattress. The curve in the lower back is accentuated. This puts pressure on spinal nerves, soft tissue, and joints. You could wake up with a very sore, stiff back.

If your head tends to hang forward, the last thing you want to do is sleep with two or three pillows lifting your head in front of your shoulders all night. Your neck should stay in a neutral position, level with your spine. When you're lying on your back, your face should point toward the ceiling. Your head should not be pushed forward or allowed to roll back, making the neck too arched and the chin jut forward.

The goal is to sleep with one thin, flat pillow that allows correct alignment. If you are used to sleeping on your back with several pillows, take one pillow away at a time so you can gradually get used to the new height.

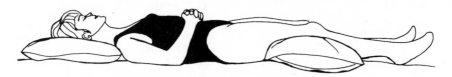

Placing pillows for sleeping on your back

Sleeping on Your Stomach

Sleeping on your stomach can be extremely hard on your neck and lower back. You have to turn your head to one side or the other, which puts a lot of pressure on the neck. Stomach sleeping allows the lower back to sag into the mattress.

If you are one of those people who can *only* sleep on their stomach, place a small pillow or rolled-up towel under your abdomen to prevent the lower back from sagging down. For even greater back relief, sleep with one knee bent toward your chest. Make sure the pillow under your head is as flat as possible so your neck doesn't have to arch as well as twist to one side.

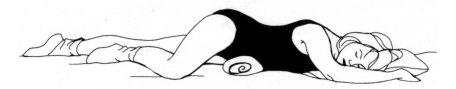

A small pillow or rolled-up towel can prevent your lower back
from sagging.

Buying a Mattress

You need a new mattress if one or more of the following is true.

- Your current mattress is more than ten years old and hasn't been flipped or turned every couple of months.

- Your mattress has lumps or sags into the middle.

- You can feel the springs or coils.

- You continually wake up with a sore, stiff back or neck.

- You roll into your partner during the night.

When you're buying a mattress, don't be shy—lie down on the models you're considering and stay in your most common sleep position for at least fifteen minutes. Select a mattress that is comfortable for you. Firm mattresses usually support the spine better, but whether the mattress is extra firm, firm, or medium soft is a matter of personal preference. A mattress that is too soft will let your body sag, causing you to wake up with aches and pains. Going from a soft mattress to a firm one will take some getting used to, and your back may be sore for the first week. Soon your body will get used to it, however, and in the long run your spine will be better supported while you

Pillow Talk

There are many kinds of pillows on the market today—rolls in all different shapes and sizes, contoured pillows, pillows stuffed with down and synthetics. Your pillow's job is to keep your neck in neutral and your head level with your spine. It should not push your head forward, allow your neck to arch, or tilt your head to the left or right.

- Side sleepers need firm pillows to fill the wide gap between the neck and mattress.

- Back sleepers need soft pillows that allow the head to sink in, so it's not pushed too far forward.

- Stomach sleepers need a thin, flat pillow or no pillow at all.

- Contoured pillows are especially designed to support the neck whether you sleep on your back or your side. They have an indentation in the middle so the head is not pushed forward. They are raised on the ends, to support the neck if the person rolls onto either side. If you tend to change position during the night, a contoured pillow is a good choice.

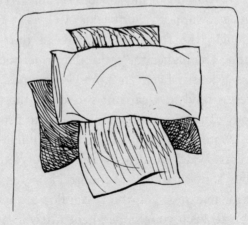

If you rest, read, or watch TV in bed, you don't want to thrust your head forward. Instead, stack up the pillows to raise your torso from the waist.

sleep. If your current mattress is too soft, but otherwise still good, you can add support by placing a three-quarters-of-an-inch-thick piece of plywood between the mattress and the box spring.

Placing a mattress topper on a firm mattress can give you the best of both worlds: comfort and firm support. The least expensive type is an "egg crate" mattress cover. A series of raised ridges distributes the pressure on body parts, allows better circulation, and keeps you cooler by allowing air to pass below you. Also available, for considerably more money, are toppers made of feathers and lambskin.

In the stores, you'll find three basic types of mattresses: innerspring, foam, and water beds. Innerspring mattresses contain coiled springs. Ask about the coil thickness. A lower gauge, which means the coils are made from thicker wire, will provide firmer support. Next, find out the number of coils or springs. A full-size bed should have at least 300; a queen-size bed at least 375, and a king-size bed at least 475. Lean over the mattress and press the palms of your hands into the surface. If you can feel the coils or springs with your hands, your body will feel them, too, and this will not be a comfortable mattress.

If you find springs uncomfortable, try a foam mattress. The right type can support your back as well as any other. However, to be firm enough, the foam should have a thirty-four-pound compression ratio. The higher the ratio, the firmer the feel. A high-quality foam has a density between 2.6 and 3 pounds per cubic foot. Foam mattresses tend to wear out sooner, as the pressure and heat of your body can change the foam's ability to provide support.

Water beds can practically eliminate uncomfortable pressure points. Water-filled beds conform to your exact shape and can give your body customized support. However, if there's not enough water in the mattress, your body can flop around, making it nearly impossible to keep your spine aligned. If you use a water bed, make sure it's filled enough to give good support.

To make your new mattress last longer (except water beds), flip and turn it every couple of months.

thirteen

Lifting Safely

Think about all the things you lift in a day: groceries, children, suitcases, vacuum cleaner, laundry basket, garbage, tools, furniture. . . . Perhaps your job involves lifting: roof shingles, furniture, mail, groceries, hospital patients. . . . Do you just reach out and hoist the load? In a quick second, you can hurt your back and cause yourself much misery. You need to stop and think about how you are lifting.

Lifting puts tremendous pressure on your vertebrae, and the way that you lift an object makes a huge difference. According to Dr. I. A. Kapandji, in his book *The Physiology of the Joints,* lifting a twenty-pound object with your knees flexed and trunk vertical exerts about 300 pounds of force on the vertebrae. Lifting the same weight while keeping the knees straight and bending over from the waist exerts about *560 pounds* on the spine.

To protect your back, learn and practice good lifting techniques. If you do a lot of lifting in your work or daily life, you should also do exercises to strengthen your abdominal muscles. Strong abs can reduce compression of the disks in your spine by as much as 50 percent.

Lifting Techniques

To keep your back working smoothly, you need to lift objects correctly. Safe lifting techniques can save your back from accidental strain and overload.

- Before you lift something, always judge its weight by pushing it with your foot. If it seems too heavy, divide the load or get someone to help you. Never carry anything you can't manage with ease.

- *Never* try to pick something up when your torso is twisted. *Lifting while the spine is twisted causes the majority of lifting injuries.* Instead, turn to face the object. Be sure your knees and torso are facing in the same direction.

- Get as close to the object as possible. The closer you are, the less strain there will be on the spine.

- Never bend from your waist. Bend your knees and hips instead. This lets the large muscles in your legs do most of the work. Bending from your waist to lift an object requires your back muscles to exert nearly twice the force.

- Tighten your abdominals as hard as you can to support your lower back before lifting or reaching for an object. When you pull your abdominals in, you increase intra-abdominal pressure, which decreases stress on your disks and joints by 50 percent. To tighten the abdominals, take a deep breath. When you exhale, pull your belly button toward your spine. Suck in as if you were trying to zip up a really tight pair of pants. Hold the abdominals in as you lift the object. Hold them in when putting the object down, too. Try not to hold your breath.

- Hold the object you've lifted close to your body as you gradually straighten your legs to a standing position. When carrying

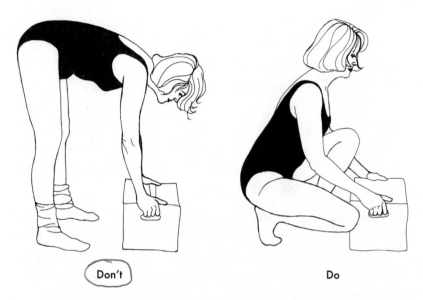

Don't   Do

an object, keep your arms close to your rib cage. The further away from your body you hold a weight, the more the disks of the spine are compressed and the more the muscles have to work.

- If you need to turn while holding the object, for example to place it onto a table, turn your feet instead of your back. Keeping your torso straight, pivot on the balls of your feet. This way your whole body turns without your spine twisting.

- When reaching for objects overhead, the same rules apply. Get as close to the object as possible. Face the object so your torso can be straight and not twisted and pull your abdominal muscles tight before you reach. Never lift a heavy object higher than your waist.

Lifting Tips

Many a person has toppled over with back pain after shoveling snow, raking the leaves, moving into a new house, even hoisting a heavy suitcase. These tips will help you lift things safely.

- Buy luggage with wheels. Don't try to carry heavy suitcases through the airport. It is almost impossible to balance the weight of a heavy suitcase evenly, and one side of your body ends up carrying the entire load.

- Try not to carry overloaded shopping bags. They place too much stress on your back, elbows, knees, and feet. Instead of carrying one very heavy shopping bag, distribute the groceries between two shopping bags, preferably with handles. Carry one in each hand.

- Moving heavy furniture can ruin your back. If possible, hire a professional mover.

- When vacuuming, never bend or twist your spine. When moving the wand forward or from side to side, use your leg muscles instead of your back—bend your knees slightly and shift your weight from one foot to another. Keep your arm close to your body rather than reaching to cover as much ground as possible.

- When raking leaves, bend your knees and place one foot forward; change the front foot often. Move forward or backward, shifting your weight from foot to foot, and dragging the leaves with the rake as you move. Don't reach too far in front of you with the rake.

- Shoveling snow can be extremely tough on the back. Take small steps; the job will take longer, but your back will be safer. Bend your knees when scooping. Before lifting the shovel filled with snow, tighten your abs to support your back. The further you try to throw the snow, the more you'll strain your back. Trade sides every few minutes. If you can afford it, a small snow thrower will make the job easier and save lots of wear and tear on your muscles and joints. Or hire a plow to take care of the driveway.

fourteen

Good Posture for Sports and Workouts

Working out or playing a sport can improve your posture by strengthening and stretching the muscles in your back, chest, abdomen, and legs. Regular aerobic and strengthening exercises can help your posture while they're making your heart and bones strong, increasing your oxygen flow, keeping your weight healthy, and reducing stress.

However, sports and workouts can strain, and even injure, your spine, joints, and muscles if you are not correctly aligned while you're doing them. If your upper back is curved too far forward, you can hurt your neck, upper back, or shoulders. If your lower back is swayed, you can have knee, hip, or lower-back injuries. If you don't consciously align yourself during athletic activity, you can wind up with a muscle pull, tendon tear, joint injury, or back pain.

Good alignment is key. If you practice good posture, you'll not only reduce your chances of injury, but will enhance your athletic performance. You will have more grace, power, and breathing capacity.

Posture and Biking

Biking is great aerobic exercise, but it's crucial that you choose the right bike and adjust it correctly.

- Select a bike frame that is the right size for your height and weight.

- Adjust the seat so that when the pedal is farthest away from you, your leg is fully extended but your knee isn't locked back.

- Most important for good posture, adjust the handlebars so you don't have to lean far forward. It is better for your back to be sitting upright. Racing bikes with curled-down handlebars encourage a head-forward position, hunched upper back, and rounded shoulders. Plus, to see in front, you have to arch your neck. Mountain bikes and hybrids with straighter handlebars are better designed for the back. Many bike stores sell attachments to raise the grips of the handlebars.

Posture and Golf

Lower-back pain is the most common complaint among golfers. This is because swinging the club causes the spine to twist forcefully (up to one hundred miles per hour). To help prevent injury, do exercises to strengthen your abdominals, because they will provide the best protection for your lower back.

Each time you follow through on a swing, you twist severely to one side. If you always swing to the left, the right side of your abdominal muscles will grow weaker, and the left side will grow tighter and more developed. To help prevent muscular imbalances, which will affect your spine, spend more time on exercises that will strengthen the weaker side and stretch the tighter side. The *Well-Balanced Golfer* exercise is a good one.

Be mindful of your posture when you swing. Keep your back as straight as possible. Bend at the hips and knees. Control your trunk motion and make sure you shift your weight correctly during the swing so that more power is generated by your hips and legs. If you can, check your posture with a professional. Poor form will eventually cause aches and pains.

When carrying your golf bag, make sure the weight is evenly distributed across your back. Occasionally switch shoulders. Before lifting the bag, pull your abdominals in tightly to support the lower back. You might want to invest in a golf bag with wheels on the bottom, which can save your back a lot of stress and strain.

Well-Balanced Golfer

Prevents muscular imbalances caused by a golf swing.

1. Lie on the floor on your back, bend your knees, and place your feet on the floor about eighteen inches from your bottom. Place both hands behind your head. Tighten your abdominals.

2. If you always swing to the left, slowly lift your left shoulder and your right knee toward each other. Hold for a slow count of five as you pull your belly button into your spine. Release. Do the opposite if you swing to the right.

3. Repeat ten to twenty times.

Posture and Tennis

When playing tennis, squash, or handball, you have to be ready to move quickly in any direction at any moment. This requires very flexible hips. You can increase the range of motion of the hips by stretching your hips, quads, and hamstrings. Keeping these muscles stretched and flexible will reduce the chance of injury and increase your power and agility. See the exercises in chapter 7.

If you always swing your racquet to the same side, one side of your torso will become tight and contracted, the other weak and stretched. Practice the *Sink Stretch* (page 67) and the *Well-Balanced Golfer* (page 125).

Though you will have to twist and turn, try to avoid sudden or jerky motions.

Posture and Running

Running and jogging pound the body against hard road surfaces over and over again. This can injure the knees, ankles, hips, back, shins, Achilles tendons, and/or calf muscles. When running or jogging, you can reduce the shock to the body by striking the ground heel first. Roll from the heel to the little toe. Then roll from the outside to the inside of the foot and push off with the big toe. Keep your abdominal muscles pulled in to support your lower back.

Make sure your rib cage is lifted and your head is pulled back over your shoulders. Don't lead with your head or chest. Holding a balanced posture while running will work more muscles in your abdomen and upper body.

Runners need to stretch their hamstrings, quads, and Achilles tendons. See the stretches in chapter 7. To stretch the Achilles tendon, do the *High-Heel Blues* (page 83).

Posture and Weight Lifting

Most gyms and health clubs have a variety of state-of-the-art weight machines designed to keep your body in the correct position while you strengthen particular muscle groups. Gyms usually have fitness trainers who can help you begin a safe and effective program.

Proper alignment is essential when using strength training machines because poor form can set you up for joint and muscle injury. Here are some ways you can make your workouts at the gym safe and effective.

- Most weight machines are constructed to hold your body in the correct position while lifting. The joint that you will be moving should be lined up with a hinge on the machine. Each time you use the machine, adjust the seat pads and other components to fit the size of your body. Before you use a machine for the first time, a fitness trainer should determine the settings for you. Write them down.

- The trainer can also help you determine the amount of weight you should be lifting. Your maximum is the amount of weight you can lift just once. Most people build up to working at 70 to 80 percent of their maximum strength. Start with low weights (50 to 60 percent of your maximum) until you get the hang of each machine.

- Warm up for five to ten minutes with light aerobic activity like cycling or walking on the treadmill.

- Whatever machine you use, always keep your head directly over your shoulders. Keep your rib cage lifted, your shoulder blades pulled back.

- Always tighten your abdominals before pushing or pulling the weight.

- If a padded backrest is provided for your back and head, use it. Sit tall with your back and head resting against the pad. This will keep your torso and head aligned.

- If you find that your shoulders hunch toward your ears while using a machine, raise the seat slightly. Always keep your shoulders squared and pressed away from your ears.

- Do two sets of eight to ten repetitions. Rest for one minute between the sets.

- Do the exercises slowly. There should be a three-second rest between each repetition.

- Always exhale when you pull the weights toward you or push them away from you.

- Don't hold your breath, as this increases the pressure in your chest, abdomen, and head.

- Don't lock your knees or elbows. This puts too much pressure on the joints, and can lead to injury.

- Drink water before, during, and after using machines. Even slight dehydration can affect the quality of your workout.

- Cool down afterward. Ask the trainer for appropriate stretches.

Good posture is also important if you use aerobic machines like StairMasters and treadmills. Many is the time I've seen people working really hard, but leaning forward to hold onto the handrails for dear life. They're reinforcing bad posture: forward head, slumped upper back. Instead, align yourself:

- Keep your head over your shoulders.

- Lift your rib cage.

Choosing an Athletic Shoe

Good athletic shoes that fit properly will help prevent injuries.

- Choose a shoe with cushioned insoles that will absorb shock and prevent the jarring of your joints. Replace the shoes (or insoles) when the insoles no longer spring back into shape after each step, even if the other parts of the shoes are still in good shape.

- Match your shoe to your activity. There are shoes designed to stabilize the foot and reduce the risk of injury during particular sports, including walking, running, aerobic dancing, and racquet sports.

- The upper part of the shoe should be flexible, but should also support the foot during movement.

- When selecting a size, stand on one foot at a time, wiggle your toes, and walk or run around the store a bit.

- The shoe has to be wide enough that the widest part of your foot fits comfortably. Shop late in the day, because feet swell during the day.

- When trying on shoes, wear the same kind of socks you will when exercising.

- If you get a pain across the top of your foot, your laces may be too tight. Loosen them to restore circulation.

- Lengthen your midsection.

- Pull in your abs.

You'll not only be helping your posture, but you'll burn more calories, since you'll be using more muscles.

Posture and Walking

Walking is an excellent low-impact exercise. To make it a total body workout, always lift your rib cage up, pull your shoulder blades back, and press your shoulders away from your ears. If you tighten your abdominals while walking, the opposing movements of your arms and legs will help strengthen them.

f i f t e e n

Eating for Stronger Muscles and Bones

The foods you eat can help strengthen your muscles and bones. I'm not talking about megavitamins or exotic supplements, but good basic nutrition, with special attention to some minerals that are particularly important for good posture: potassium, magnesium, and calcium.

Healthy Choices

For good health in general, your diet should be low in saturated fats and high in lean meats (or other whole protein), whole grains, fruits, and vegetables. These foods, which reduce the risk of cancer, heart disease, and other health problems, will help your muscles and bones, too.

You also need a moderate amount of protein, which provides the building blocks for muscle tissues and bones. However, if you eat more protein than your body needs, it will just be converted into body fat. It's not true, despite the claims of protein drinks and bars, that eating lots of protein will build big muscles. According to Dr. Miriam Nelson of the School of Nutrition Science at Tufts Univer-

> ### How Much Protein Do You Need?
>
> To figure out how many grams of protein you should have each day, multiply your weight in kilograms (weight in pounds times 2.2) by .8. For example, if you weigh 150 pounds, you need 150 times 2.2 times .8 grams per day: 54 grams of protein.
>
> One ounce of meat has about 7 grams of protein, and one cup of dairy foods has about 8 grams.

sity, our bodies rebuild and replace about one pound of muscle tissue each day. About three-quarters of the necessary protein is recycled in the process. So we need at least one-fourth of a pound (four ounces) of protein daily from our diet to help us maintain and repair our muscles.

According to the American Dietetic Association, between 10 and 15 percent of your calories should come from protein. For the average woman, that's about fifty grams of protein; for the average man, sixty-three grams. It's easy to get that much—two cups of skim milk, a cup of low-fat yogurt, and a small chicken breast will do it. Eat a small amount of protein with each meal.

A low-fat diet (along with regular exercise) will also help you keep your weight at a healthy level. Extra pounds put stress on the weight-bearing joints, including the spine. Extra weight in the abdominal area (an "apple-shaped" figure) can pull the lower back into an arch.

Potassium for Strong Muscles

For strong muscles, you need potassium. This mineral is necessary for synthesizing muscle protein. The U.S. dietary goal for potassium is two thousand milligrams per day for an average, healthy adult or child over ten. (The dietary goal for a nutrient, also called the Recommended Dietary Allowance or R.D.A., is set by the U.S. Food and Nutrition Board, National Academy of Sciences, and National Research Council.) The average American gets only one

BEST-CHOICE FOODS

This chart can help you remember to include the foods that are nutritional superstars in your diet. For superior nutrition, choose foods you really like from each category and include them in your weekly diet.

Vegetables	Fruit	Beans	Grains
artichoke	apples	black beans	amaranth
asparagus	apricots	black-eyed peas	barley
avocado	bananas	chickpeas	brown rice
broccoli	blackberries	kidney beans	buckwheat
Brussels sprouts	blueberries	lentils	bulgar
cabbage	cantaloupe	lima beans	millet
carrots	cherries	navy beans	oats
cauliflower	dried apricots	pink beans	quinoa
collard greens	grapefruits	pinto beans	rye
corn	grapes	soybeans	whole rye
endive	honeydews	white beans	wild rice
green peas	kiwis		whole wheat
kale	mangos		
kohlrabi	nectarines		
mushrooms	oranges		
okra	peaches		
parsley	pears		
parsnips	persimmons		
red pepper	pineapples		
romaine lettuce	plums		
rutabaga	pomegranates		
snow peas	prunes		
spinach	raspberries		
sweet potato/yam	star fruits		
Swiss chard	strawberries		
tomatoes	tangerines		
white potatoes	watermelons		
winter squash			

thousand milligrams per day. Many experts agree that potassium intake, from food, should really be thirty-five hundred to five thousand milligrams per day.

Potassium should be derived only from food, *never* from a pill unless prescribed by a physician. This should not be too difficult, as it is abundant in many fruits and vegetables. You should eat between five and nine servings of fruits and vegetables each day.

Americans come up short on potassium because we don't eat enough fruits and vegetables, and also because there is way too much salt in our diet. A high-salt diet causes potassium to be lost in the urine. Processed, refined, baked, canned, and packaged foods, and frozen dinners and restaurant foods, are loaded with salt. Potassium can also be depleted by prolonged diarrhea, stress, excessive sweating, vomiting, and the use of diuretics.

Reducing Sodium

Many people find that it's easier to get more potassium in their diets than to get the sodium out. We need only five hundred milligrams of sodium daily to maintain proper health, but the average American easily consumes five thousand to eight thousand milligrams per day. The American Dietetic Association recommends a maximum of twenty-four hundred milligrams of sodium per day, or about one teaspoon. A whopping 75 percent of all dietary salt comes from processed, packaged, and refined foods. To lower your intake:

- Check the sodium content of packaged foods by reading the labels. Many processed foods, including most canned vegetables and soups, are high in sodium. Try not to purchase foods containing added salt, sodium, or compounds like monosodium glutamate (MSG).

- When you eat in restaurants, ask for unsalted food. Send the order back if it comes salted anyway. Many restaurants now prepare low-sodium dishes. Limit fast-food meals, since they are loaded with salt.

- Experiment with lots of herbs and spices instead of using table salt in recipes.

> **Foods High in Sodium**
>
> **Meats:** bacon, bologna, canned meats, ham, hot dogs, salami, sausage.
>
> **Canned fish:** salmon, sardines, tuna.
>
> **Snacks:** cheeses, crackers, dips, pretzels, salted nuts.
>
> **Condiments:** catsup, mayonnaise, mustard, olives, pickles, relish, salad dressing.
>
> **Seasonings:** barbecue sauce, boullion cubes, celery salt, chili sauce, cooking wine, garlic salt, meat tenderizers, monosodium glutamate (MSG), onion salt, tamari sauce, smoke flavoring, soy sauce, Worcestershire sauce.

- Many people have found fresh lemon juice to be especially helpful when trying to kick the salt habit. Lemon juice acts on the same region of your tongue that salt does—it sort of tricks your tongue into thinking it's having salt. Also, by squeezing fresh lemon juice over vegetables and meats, instead of salt, you'll be decreasing sodium and increasing vitamin C, potassium, and folic acid. Also, the vitamin C makes it easier for your body to absorb more iron from the food you are eating. Buy a few fresh lemons and keep them in your refrigerator. Cut a wedge as needed.

Magnesium for Muscles and Bones

While too *much* sodium depletes your potassium, too *little* magnesium does the same. Magnesium helps cells store potassium until they need it. It also aids bone growth and is necessary for the proper functioning of the nerves and muscles. In fact, magnesium is responsible for more biochemical reactions in the body than any other mineral, but unfortunately is one of the most overlooked nutrients. Make sure you get enough in your diet.

A deficiency in magnesium can cause muscle spasms or charley horses in the lower legs. If you suffer from leg spasms or muscular tension, consume several foods rich in magnesium each day. Magnesium can ease spasms within minutes of absorption.

Millions of Americans don't get enough magnesium in their diets because they don't eat enough beans, whole grains, and dark green leafy vegetables like kale, collards, and spinach. The Recommended Dietary Allowance (RDA) for magnesium is 400 milligrams for adults and 450 milligrams for pregnant, breast-feeding, or postmenopausal women. Most people don't come close. The body's supply of magnesium can be depleted by vomiting, diarrhea, use of laxatives, alcohol consumption, diet pills, diuretics, birth control pills, or a diet high in fats, refined foods, and stress.

If you won't eat the foods richest in magnesium, then you may need to buy a magnesium supplement. Choose one that contains magnesium oxide. If you are prone to diarrhea, choose a magnesium citrate supplement. Take one tablet containing two hundred to four hundred milligrams of magnesium daily.

Calcium for Strong Bones

Calcium is essential for strong bones. Bones store most of the body's calcium, which is also needed by the body for other purposes.

Every day that you do not consume enough calcium, your body will take what it needs from your bones. Day after day, week after week, year after year, and decade after decade of calcium deficiency can easily lead to osteoporosis: thin, fragile bones.

The Daily Value for calcium was recently increased to one thousand milligrams per day. During pregnancy and lactation, women need twelve hundred milligrams per day. Postmenopausal women should have fifteen hundred milligrams of calcium daily.

The richest source of calcium is nonfat or low-fat milk and dairy products. Other sources include canned salmon with bones, tofu, broccoli, parsley, watercress, almonds, asparagus, brewer's yeast, blackstrap molasses, cabbage, carob figs, filberts, prunes, sesame seeds, kelp, mustard greens, oats, and whole wheat.

If you don't get enough calcium in your diet, then you need to take a supplement. Calcium carbonate, the most common form, is a good choice, but you have to take it with meals so that it can be absorbed well. Supplements containing calcium citrate are most easily absorbed, but are also usually more expensive.

Your body will probably not be able to absorb doses larger than five hundred to six hundred milligrams at a time, so split your daily dose over two or three meals. Take one of your calcium pills before bed. It is at night, when you are asleep, that your body will take calcium from your bones if there is not enough in your bloodstream. Taking a calcium supplement before bed will eliminate your body's need to take it from your bones.

Look at the label of your calcium supplement. If it has the letters

> ### How Much Calcium Should You Supplement?
>
> To figure out how many milligrams of supplement to take, start by figuring out how much calcium you usually get from food. One cup of milk or yogurt (the most common sources) contains about 300 milligrams of calcium. If you regularly have two servings, you are getting 600 milligrams a day. If you need 1,000 milligrams a day, you need 400 milligrams from supplements.

"USP," the supplement meets the U.S. Pharmacopoeia's strict standard for dissolution, and your supplement will dissolve. Try the vinegar test as well. Place one of your supplements in a cup of ordinary white vinegar and let it sit. If the supplement doesn't dissolve within thirty minutes, you may not be getting any benefit from it. Some supplements won't even dissolve if you leave them in the vinegar overnight, which means they are useless to you because they'll just pass through your digestive tract whole and the nutrients won't be available for absorption.

Vitamin D helps your body absorb calcium. Vitamin D stimulates the production of the protein carriers—boats, if you will—that carry calcium molecules through the bloodstream to their various destinations. The RDA is four hundred international units a day. An eight-ounce glass of fortified milk contains one hundred units. Your body manufactures vitamin D when your skin is exposed to sunlight, but most people don't get enough of the vitamin without drinking fortified milk or taking a supplement, especially in winter when they're covered up.

Signs of a Good Supplement

It would be ideal to get all of our nutrients from fresh, healthy food, but most diets are less than ideal. If your diet isn't all it should be, a balanced, well-made multivitamin and mineral supplement can fill some of the nutritional gaps. The supplement's label should state that it contains 100 percent of the U.S. RDA (United States Recommended Dietary Allowance) for all the vitamins and minerals that the National Research Council has said are needed by the human body for health. If a product doesn't have them, don't buy it. Specifically check for:

1. *Similar percentages of the eight B vitamins.* These work better together than separately. When one or two B vitamins are supplied in much higher amounts than others are, it throws the balance out of whack. Beware of supplements that have

huge percents of the cheaper vitamins (B1, B2, B3) and much smaller amounts of others (folic acid, B6, B12).

2. *At least 100 percent RDA of biotin, a B vitamin that's vital for health.* Because it is the most expensive B vitamin, many supplements have far less.

3. *One hundred percent RDA of both zinc and copper.* Some supplements skimp on zinc.

You will probably have to buy a calcium/magnesium supplement to go along with your multivitamin. Calcium and magnesium are very big molecules. If a multivitamin/mineral were to include enough of these two minerals, the tablet would have to be the size of a horse pill. Get calcium citrate or carbonate with magnesium oxide. A good formula has two parts calcium to one part magnesium. For example, if the supplement contains 500 milligrams of calcium, it should have 250 milligrams of magnesium.

Taking supplements should never be used as an excuse to eat poorly. Look at it this way: When you eat a piece of fruit or vegetable, you get small amounts of thousands of compounds that contribute to your health. When you take a supplement, you only get a handful. Eat as well as you can—fill your diet with fruits, vegetables, grains, lean meats, nuts, and seeds and use a balanced, well-made supplement to fill in the nutritional gaps.

Vitamins, Minerals, and Trace Minerals with an Established U.S. RDA	
Vitamin A	Vitamin C
Vitamin B$_1$ (thiamine)	Vitamin D
	Vitamin E
Vitamin B$_2$ (riboflavin)	Calcium
	Magnesium
Vitamin B$_3$ (niacin)	Boron
	Chromium
Vitamin B$_5$ (pantothenic acid)	Copper
	Iodine
	Iron
Vitamin B$_6$ (pyndoxine)	Manganese
	Phosphorus
Vitamin B$_{12}$ (cobalamine)	Selenium
	Zinc
Biotin (a B vitamin)	Molybdenum
Folic acid (folate; a B vitamin)	

4

Special Concerns

Help for the
Baby *Backache* Blues

Good posture becomes very important when you are pregnant or have a new baby. Many common discomforts of pregnancy are linked to poor posture: an aching lower back, tight upper back, rounded shoulders, sciatic nerve pain, even breathlessness. The problems don't stop after the birth—in fact, backaches become even more likely.

The weight of the baby, whether it's inside or out, puts an extra load on your spine. The mother's muscles have to support this unaccustomed load. And since the weight isn't centered over the mother's center of gravity, it can pull the alignment out of whack, especially that of the lower back. At the same time, hormones are loosening the mother's muscles and joints and making them vulnerable. No wonder the baby backache blues are so common!

During Pregnancy

During pregnancy, as at other times, lower-back pain occurs when the lower spine has an exaggerated curve. The weight of the growing baby in the uterus pulls the lower part of the spine forward

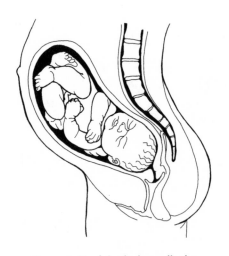

The weight of the baby pulls the lower spine forward.

into an extreme arch, causing pressure and irritation in the joints, disks, nerves, and muscles. The spine also has to support more weight than usual.

Most pregnant women try to compensate for the load in front by leaning their upper body back, creating even more pressure in the lower back.

Allowing the upper body to slump forward because of fatigue or bad habit makes it even more difficult to breathe deeply than it already is. The growing fetus will decrease the height of the lung cavity by as much as four centimeters, so your lungs need all the room they can get.

Slumping presses the rib cage down on the stomach, too. Like the lungs, the stomach is already short on space. It's being pressed between the growing uterus and the diaphragm. Stomach acid can be pushed into the esophagus, causing heartburn.

By standing and sitting properly, and by doing posture exercises, you can help avoid these common discomforts of pregnancy. However, it's important to stretch gently and to change or skip exercises that might put too much strain on your joints. During pregnancy and for six months afterward, you can easily injure your knees, ankles, hips, or back. All your joints are looser and less stable than usual because they're being affected by the hormones your body is producing to loosen the ligaments in the pelvis so the baby can pass through at birth. Your tendons and muscles are looser, too.

You should also skip exercises that require you to lie on your back. The American College of Obstetricians and Gynecologists

(ACOG) says that women should not exercise on their backs after the fourth month of pregnancy because the heavy uterus could press on a major vein and reduce the flow of blood from the legs back to the heart. Less blood could reach your brain, causing light-headedness or dizziness. Eventually, less blood could reach the fetus. Instead, choose exercises done against a wall, standing, or sitting.

When participating in any aerobic activity, do not let your pulse rate go higher than 140 beats per minute (23 to 24 beats per 10 second count). The concern is that you'll overheat. You can sweat to lose heat but your fetus cannot, which could lead to neural tube defects during the first trimester. Never work to the point of being breathless or dripping with sweat.

Some women in the later stages of pregnancy develop carpal tunnel syndrome—numbness and tingling in their hands and fingers. If you do, skip the resistance exercises and wall push-ups.

Check with your doctor before doing this or any other exercise program.

If you keep these cautions in mind, you can safely and effectively improve and protect your posture during pregnancy. In fact, considering the problems poor posture can cause for you, posture improvement has never been more important than now. Here is a posture program for pregnancy:

- Practice *One Minute to Better Posture* (page 13).

- To help prevent lower-back aches, do the *Standing Pelvic Tilt* (page 62).

- Remember to keep your knees soft when you're standing (stiff, locked-back knees increase the curve in your lower back).

- To stop the slump, do exercises from chapter 5, and also the *Shoulder Unrounder* and *Elbow Press* in chapter 6.

- To keep your abdominal muscles as strong as possible, do the *Abdomen Tighteners* (pages 68–69) often throughout the day.

- Don't do any exercises in which you would lie flat on your back.

- Avoid bending from the waist. Lower your body by bending your knees and hips while keeping your back straight.

- Be mindful of how you stand, sit, move, and even sleep.

The *Second* Nine Months

The baby's out, so why does your back ache more than ever? During pregnancy, your abdominal muscles stretched to twice their original length. After delivery, they don't automatically shrink back. As long as the abdominals remain loose, they can't support your lower back, and it sags into an exaggerated arch that puts pressure on nerves, joints, and soft tissues.

Backaches are also caused by lifting, lowering, and carrying the baby. You're also lugging a lot of stuff around: baby, baby carrier, diaper bag, plus your purse. Your lower back really needs the support of strong abdominal muscles.

Strengthening your abs will also help you get your waistline back. During the first few months of pregnancy, the bottom three ribs flare out in anticipation of your growing baby. After you deliver, the ribs remain slightly flared unless eased back in. Since the abdominals are attached to the bottom of the rib cage, as you re-strengthen them, they will pull the ribs back in, and you'll have a waist again.

Another common postpartum problem area is the upper back. New moms spend much of their time holding, cradling, and nursing their new baby with their upper back and shoulders rounded forward. Often, they develop a lot of upper-back discomfort, including "hot spots" between their shoulder blades.

You can begin exercising as soon as it feels comfortable, usually after two or three weeks, but check first with your doctor.

Since you probably don't have a chunk of time to set aside for exercise, your best bets are the anytime/anywhere exercises (see chapter 3). Some of them can even be done while you're holding or feeding your baby.

Be sure you do the exercises that strengthen your abdominal muscles. Next, focus on stopping the slump. Practice *One Minute to Better Posture* and the exercises in the chapters on the upper back and the shoulders. Any of the exercises in the book will benefit you. Do stretches carefully and moderately, since your ligaments can remain loose for up to six months after the birth. Don't be discouraged if the results aren't immediate. It took nine months for your body to get this way!

How to Lift a Baby

To protect your back, pay attention to the position of your body when you are feeding, changing, and carrying your baby. The new father should use safe lifting techniques, too.

- *Carrying your baby.* Many mothers and fathers lean back to compensate for the child's weight. This puts pressure on the lower back and results in pain and discomfort. When holding or carrying your baby, make sure your hips are tucked under (pelvis is in neutral, see page 59), abdominals pulled in, and torso held erect. Avoid always carrying your baby on the same side. Switch sides often, or try to carry your baby in front so that the weight is evenly distributed. Baby backpacks center the weight evenly across your back, but be sure not to tip your torso back or too far forward to compensate for the extra weight you're carrying. Snugglies allow you to carry your baby in front, evenly centered. Your baby can hear your heartbeat and be within your sight, too. Some slings can put too much pressure on one shoulder, but others, I've been told, are really comfortable. There are many different kinds of baby-carrying devices on the market—try them out, if possible, in the store before buying one.

- *Baths.* For the first six months, bathe your baby in the kitchen sink rather than bending over a tub. (While you're standing there, you can work in a Pelvic Tilt, Abdomen Tightener, or Buttock Clencher.)

- *Feeding.* When breast-feeding or bottle-feeding, instead of rounding your upper back forward to reach the baby, bring the baby up to you. If you're breast-feeding, turn the baby completely toward you (you'll be tummy to tummy). Rest the baby's weight on some pillows in your lap, rather than fully with your arms.

- *Car seats.* Car seats are safe for babies, but treacherous for their parents' backs. When you put the baby in a car seat, you have to twist your torso and hold the baby's full weight with your arms stretched out. This puts a tremendous strain on the disks and ligaments in your back. To reduce the strain, reduce the distance you have to reach. To place an infant in a rear-facing car seat, sit on the seat next to the car seat, then place the infant in the chair. To put a child in a forward-facing seat, first tighten your abdominals to support your back, then get as close to the car seat as possible. While facing the rear of the car, place your foot inside on the rear floor so that most of your body is inside the car. You should be squatting slightly, and your torso should not be twisted.

- *Cribs.* Putting your baby into and out of a crib and taking it out again can be hazardous to your back if you don't lift and bend with caution. Remember that for the first six months after delivery, your back is vulnerable because your ligaments are still loose and your abdominals are still stretched. Raise the crib mattress to the highest level for the first six months so that you don't have to lean over so far. Before lifting your baby, always support your back by tightening your abdominal muscles and keeping your pelvis in neutral. Keep your knees slightly bent as you lift. Avoid twisting your back when lifting the baby up or placing the baby back down.

seventeen

Osteoporosis and Posture

A broken hip or a curved upper spine affects so many older women that many people think they're inevitable parts of aging. These are not normal, but rather are signs of a medical disorder, osteoporosis—porous, weak, fragile bones. Osteoporosis leads to a fracture for half of women over age fifty. These fractures, most often in the wrist, hip, or spine, are not only painful, but can limit a woman's activities and independence.

Osteoporosis affects men also. But men start out with thicker bones than women so it takes them longer to be in danger of fracturing, usually not until around the age of eighty. However, men also need to consume adequate calcium to keep themselves healthy.

Though the effects of osteoporosis are seen in older people, mostly women, the condition develops over a lifetime. People of every age can build stronger bones to help avoid this. In this chapter, you'll learn ways to help increase your bone density. If you have already been diagnosed with osteoporosis, you'll learn how to reduce your risk of fractures by improving your posture and muscle strength.

Building Stronger Bones

Though bones look like permanent structures, their tissues are constantly being removed and added. Until a person is about twenty-five, new bone cells are added faster than old bone cells are removed, so the bones become larger and denser. After thirty-five, bone is lost faster than it's added, particularly after menopause—unless the person takes steps to build bone. Decades of research have shown that there is lots you can do not only to slow bone loss, but actually increase bone density after the age of thirty-five.

If you'd like to know how your bones are holding up, talk with your doctor about a bone-density scan. It is a good idea to get a bone-density measurement before you reach menopause as a baseline for later comparison. Yearly scans will let you know if you are losing bone, remaining steady, or increasing bone density, and will be helpful if you are deciding whether to have hormone replacement therapy.

There are three ways to keep your bones strong: diet, weight-bearing exercise, and hormone replacement.

Nutrition

At every age, calcium is essential for strong bones, because it increases the density of the bones. Your body also needs calcium for other functions, including the contraction of the heart and other muscles. Every day that you do not consume enough calcium in your diet, your body has no choice but to take calcium from your bones to meet its other needs. If you don't get enough calcium in your diet, your bones become weaker and weaker year after year.

Most women get only half the recommended amount of calcium, which is one thousand to fifteen hundred milligrams daily. See chapter 15 for information on getting enough calcium. Many women should take a supplement.

You also need to get enough vitamin D, so your body can absorb the calcium. For strong bones you also need magnesium, phosphorous, and boron. To keep your bones and your whole body healthy, fill your diet with fruits, vegetables, beans, whole grains, lean meats, nuts and seeds, and nonfat dairy products (or other calcium-rich foods if you are lactose intolerant). Consuming enough calcium every day is crucial to bone health.

Weight-Bearing Exercise

To build your bones, you have to do activities that put weight on them. Walking, jogging, and weight lifting are good examples. Just as your heart and lungs become stronger with regular aerobic exercise, your bones become stronger with regular weight-bearing exercise. Research has shown that three hours of weight-bearing exercise each week can decrease bone loss by 75 percent. Exercise can even increase bone mass after menopause. No matter what your age, it is never too late to benefit from exercise.

Make weight-bearing exercise a regular part of your life. Walking is excellent for overall health and well-being. Join a walking club or enlist a neighbor to walk with you regularly. To start, walk for ten or fifteen minutes. Gradually lengthen the walk to thirty to forty-five minutes or longer.

Hormone Replacement Therapy

If a bone-density scan has shown your bones to be strong and thick, then good nutrition and weight-bearing exercise should continue to keep you healthy. If your bones are thinner than they should be, or if you are at high risk for osteoporosis, talk with your doctor when you are approaching menopause about whether or not you should take natural hormones to slow the rate of bone loss and decrease the chance of fractures. Natural hormones can alleviate menopausal symptoms such as hot flashes, vaginal dryness, and sleep disturbance.

I suggest that you investigate natural alternatives to synthetic hormones, especially natural progesterone and the natural estrogens found in soy and flaxseed. I strongly recommend the book *What Your Doctor May Not Tell You About Menopause* by Dr. John R. Lee.

Remember, you play the most essential role in protecting your bones. Stand tall, eat healthy foods, and stay active!

If You Have Osteoporosis

If you have been diagnosed with osteoporosis, your risk of bone fractures is very high, so you should check with your doctor or physical therapist before you embark on an exercise program to ensure that you don't put too much stress on your bones.

If you get the go-ahead, exercises that improve the flexibility and strength of your back can help relieve the pain of spinal fractures and reduce the chances that more will occur. When the bones have been weakened by osteoporosis, hairline cracks can occur in the vertebrae that make up the spine. Eventually, the body's weight can crush the weakened vertebra. These painful fractures cause tremendous curving of the upper spine and loss of height.

A slouched, rounded-forward posture increases the chance that a vertebra will fracture and collapse, because it puts stress on the area most likely to fracture. All of the tips, techniques, and exercises included in this book will help you stop the rounding over that occurs as you age, and will help take pressure off spinal bones.

Regularly practice the exercise *One Minute to Better Posture*. Every time you think of it, lift your rib cage, pull your shoulder blades back, and pull your belly muscles in. Also, be sure to do the *Abdomen Tighteners*, really concentrating on the breathing portion of the exercises, to help keep your rib cage mobile.

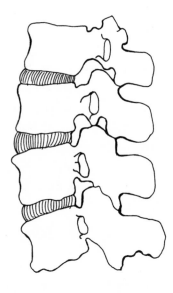 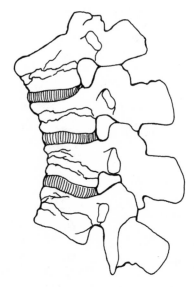

Healthy vertebrae   Vertebrae that have collapsed

By increasing the strength of your legs and the flexibility of your ankles, you'll reduce your risk of falls. Many fractures happen because older people lose their balance easily (even when making an ordinary move like turning too fast or reaching up or down), then don't have the strength to stop themselves once they start to topple. Try the exercises in chapter 8. They'll strengthen your feet and ankles and improve your flexibility.

For all of the exercises, start with three repetitions and gradually build to ten, adding one each day. If any exercise causes discomfort, omit it. For the resistance exercises, try one repetition and see how your joints feel. Choose the easier versions of exercises and always use very light resistance to begin.

Don't do exercises in which you would bend forward at the waist or twist your spine—there aren't any in this book, but you may encounter them in other exercise programs or classes.

All of the lying-down exercises should be done on your bed, because getting down to and up from the floor could be too difficult. If your upper back is too curved forward, you may need to place a thin pillow under your head so your neck doesn't have to arch in order for your head to rest against the bed.

Tips for Protecting Your Back

Proper lifting and other good body mechanics become even more important if you have osteoporosis.

- Never bend over to pick up an object. This places too much pressure on the front of the vertebrae and can lead to compression fractures of the spine. See chapter 13.

- When brushing your teeth, bend at the knees rather than the waist.

- When coughing or sneezing, place one hand on your lower back, lift your rib cage up and tighten your abdominals. This will help protect vertebrae and disks from injury caused by a sudden bend forward.

- Never bend or twist the spine when vacuuming or raking. See chapter 13.

- Don't sit too long. While sitting, circle your ankles in different directions.

- When you need to stand in place for more than a few minutes, put one of your feet up on a stool or railing.

- Try to stay as active as possible. Inactivity causes bones to weaken.

e i g h t e e n

Should You Seek Medical Help?

A 1994 study by the Agency for Health Care Policy and Research found that 90 percent of back problems resolve and heal themselves without medical intervention, and that most people resume normal activities within a month. So it's generally fine to work on back discomfort yourself rather than seek a doctor right away. However, if you have back or neck pain that occurs suddenly, or that has lasted a long time, it's a good idea to get a doctor's opinion.

Usually, sudden pain follows years of poor posture, when the person bends, lifts, or reaches. Improving posture and body mechanics (the way one sits, stands, moves, lifts) is the best way to prevent a recurrence.

Treating Minor Pain Yourself

If you have a minor backache or neck ache, your goal is to reduce the pain and inflammation. Inflammation stretches the tissues, causing more pain and interfering with healing.

- Take an anti-inflammatory pain reliever like aspirin (unless you are allergic to it) or ibuprofen. These over-the-counter drugs are just as effective as prescription muscle relaxants and have fewer side effects.

- As soon as possible after an injury, ice it down. Keep icing it for ten to twenty minutes every two hours for forty-eight hours or until the swelling subsides. You can use a frozen blue gel pack, or place ice cubes in a plastic bag, or use a bag of frozen corn kernels or peas. Wrap either in a thin towel—never apply directly to the skin.

- Rest, but only for the first day. A Finnish study published in the *New England Journal of Medicine* showed that even two days of bed rest can slow recovery by weakening the muscles. Try to go about your normal activities.

When to Seek Medical Care

You should see your doctor if you have back or neck pain and:

- You have been in an accident (a car accident or a fall).

- You feel numbness or tingling.

- There is a line of shooting pain into your buttocks or legs.

- The pain is sharp or stabbing.

- There is stiffness or a decrease in range of motion.

- You have any weakness in your ankle, big toe, hand, or fingers, or a loss of gripping power in your hand.

- A neck pain persists longer than ten days, or a stiff neck is accompanied by fever or nausea (symptoms of meningitis).

Conventional medical treatment will start with an examination by your primary care physician. The doctor will evaluate the pain and will want to rule out any serious problems, such as a fracture, dislocation, or tumor. You may have imaging studies such as an X ray, CT scan, or MRI to detect bone or soft tissue damage.

You may be referred to a specialist. If nerve damage is suspected, you'll be referred to a neurologist (a medical doctor who treats disorders of the brain, spine, and nerves) or a neurosurgeon. Orthopedists and orthopedic surgeons specialize in bones, joints, and muscles. They treat a wide range of problems, from herniated disks to traumatic injuries.

If it is suspected that you have injured a muscle or joint, your doctor may refer you to a licensed physical therapist. Look for a therapist who specializes in back and neck pain. The therapist will evaluate your posture and the source of your pain, then teach you specific exercises and stretches for your individual needs. The therapist will also show you ways to move through your daily activities as efficiently as possible while protecting your back.

Alternative Therapies

A wide range of alternative therapies places great importance on posture. You may find that one of them will help you develop better posture as well as relieve pain in your back, neck, or elsewhere. When pursuing an alternative therapy, look for a practitioner who has been trained and licensed. Tell your medical doctor that you plan to try the alternative therapy.

Chiropractic

Over two-thirds of people with back pain go to chiropractors, and the treatment has a good track record. The Agency for Health

Care Policy and Research, part of the U.S. Department of Health and Human Services, has said that chiropractic treatments can help patients with acute lower-back pain. For chronic pain, though, researchers' findings are mixed. The agency recommended that treatments be stopped if the symptoms do not improve within a month.

Chiropractors believe that most back pain is caused by misalignments (called subluxations) of the spinal bones. They manipulate the spine to restore the correct positioning of the vertebrae. Treatment should not be painful and should include exercises and education to prevent recurrence.

Bodywork

Many alternative therapies and techniques can relieve the tension and stress in muscles. The Alexander Technique teaches people to properly align the head, neck, and torso, and consciously use new and better patterns of movement. Yoga is a wonderful way to increase flexibility (but avoid poses that arch the neck and lower back: for example, the plough). There are massage therapies like Swedish massage as well as deep tissue manipulation like Rolfing. You may wish to explore some of these therapies.

Acupuncture

Acupuncture has been used as a healing art in China for over 3,000 years. The principle behind acupuncture is to balance the body's flow of energy. If the acupuncturist finds an imbalance of energy flow, he or she will place very thin sterile needles into specific meridian points. Acupuncturists believe that pain is caused by a block in energy. The fine needles restore the flow.

Most people feel nothing when the needles are inserted just below the skin. Some feel a slight sensation. Although they may sound frightening, acupuncture treatments are not painful. Most people find them comforting and relaxing. And many have found relief from aches and pains.

Acupuncturists do not have to be medical doctors, though some are, so you'll need to check if they are Certified (C.A.) or Licensed (L.Ac.) Different states have different requirements.

Index of Exercises and Stretches